Sana BEKRI
Amel LABIDI

MANAGEMENT OF MANDIBULAR TOTAL AND SUBTOTAL EDENTURES

Sana BEKRI
Amel LABIDI

MANAGEMENT OF MANDIBULAR TOTAL AND SUBTOTAL EDENTURES

ScienciaScripts

Imprint
Any brand names and product names mentioned in this book are subject to trademark, brand or patent protection and are trademarks or registered trademarks of their respective holders. The use of brand names, product names, common names, trade names, product descriptions etc. even without a particular marking in this work is in no way to be construed to mean that such names may be regarded as unrestricted in respect of trademark and brand protection legislation and could thus be used by anyone.

Cover image: www.ingimage.com

This book is a translation from the original published under ISBN 978-620-6-72562-6.

Publisher:
Sciencia Scripts
is a trademark of
Dodo Books Indian Ocean Ltd. and OmniScriptum S.R.L publishing group

120 High Road, East Finchley, London, N2 9ED, United Kingdom
Str. Armeneasca 28/1, office 1, Chisinau MD-2012, Republic of Moldova, Europe
Managing Directors: Ieva Konstantinova, Victoria Ursu
info@omniscriptum.com

Printed at: see last page
ISBN: 978-620-8-85022-7

Summary

List of abbreviations

CMC: Carboxymethylcellulose

CR/RR: Radiographic crown-to-root ratio.

DVO: Vertical dimension of occlusion.

HOPU: Prosthetically usable occlusal height.

MECT: Tissue conditioning.

N: Newton.

PAC: Complete Denture.

PACSI: Supra-Implant Complete Denture. **PACSR:** Supra-Radicular Complete Denture. **PEI:** Individual Impression Tray.

PIM: Maximum Intercuspal Position.

RC: Centric relation.

Introduction

Advances in scientific knowledge and technology have led to considerable progress in dentistry. Indeed, advances in restorative dentistry and periodontology, as well as efforts to promote oral health, have made it possible to
preserve teeth longer and in better condition. However, despite these efforts, total tooth loss remains high due to the aging population and increased life expectancy (34). This means that complete prosthetic rehabilitation remains a frequent, difficult, and demanding procedure. This difficulty is even greater in the case of complete mandibular dentures, where the support surface is generally narrow (34, 66).
As such, retention and stability, often considered insufficient by patients, are the most common complaints, particularly in cases of long-standing edentulism with advanced bone resorption (2).
Depending on the clinical situation and the economic circumstances of the patient, several options can be considered to improve the retention and stability of complete mandibular dentures.
In this book, we will detail the various means available to practitioners to optimize this prosthetic therapy. Clinical cases will be used to better illustrate our points.

OPTIMIZATION OF CONVENTIONAL COMPLETE MANDIBULAR PROSTHESES

In cases of complete mandibular edentulism, conventional complete dentures are no longer the treatment of first choice, particularly with the advent of implants; however, they remain a clinical reality for a significant number of patients, either due to fear of treatment or lack of financial resources (45).

The denture fabrication process and the quality of each step influence prosthetic stability. However, despite compliance with fabrication requirements, this treatment remains delicate and sometimes produces poor results (22, 2).

Indeed, the small support surface and the presence of the tongue and peripheral structures significantly compromise adhesion, which is an essential factor in the retention of complete removable dentures.

The practitioner must therefore remain vigilant, as managing post-prosthetic complaints can be frustrating and time-consuming after prosthetic insertion.

It is therefore essential to follow all stages of the procedure. In addition, certain therapies can improve the prosthesis (45).

1. Pre-prosthetic surgery

A complete mandibular denture requires maximum use of the anatomical areas that can optimize prosthetic support and retention. Some cases of tooth loss can hinder proper prosthetic restoration, so pre-prosthetic surgery may be necessary. Taking impressions of altered or deformed tissue can cause the prosthesis to become unstable and therefore trigger pain once the prosthesis is inserted (67, 37).

Pre-prosthetic surgery is a means of creating a better anatomical environment, which is necessary for the manufacture of a well-fitting, functional, comfortable, and aesthetic prosthesis (26).

Two objectives summarize the importance of pre-prosthetic surgery:

1. Correction of conditions that prevent optimal prosthetic function (26):

- Mucosal hyperplasia and floating ridges
- Poorly positioned frenula.
- Bony prominences and undercuts

2. Enlargement of the areas supporting the prosthesis:

- Vestibuloplasty
- Crest augmentation

1.1. Indications

1.1.1. At the mucosal level [30,21,35,73,26]

❖ ***Fibrous hyperplasia*** (30, 21)

This is a traumatic lesion in the form of folds and fibrous growths of the oral mucosa under and around the prosthetic margins that sink into the vestibule following bone resorption. It is usually located at the bottom of the anterior vestibule, the mucosal reflection areas, or on the slopes of the ridges (Figure 1). It is a pathological response to chronic irritation.

The decision to operate depends on the volume, location, and the patient's consent ( ).

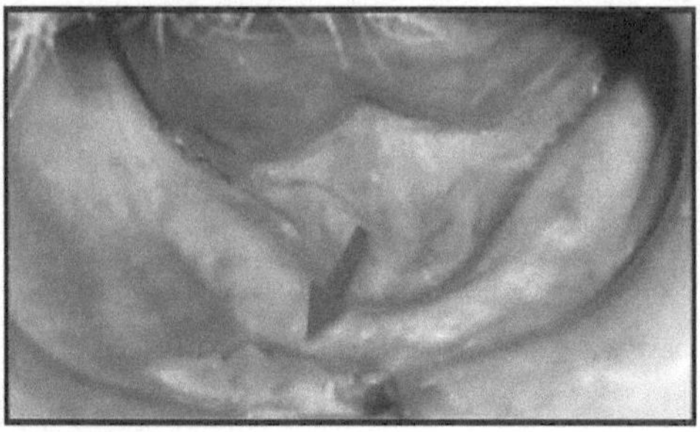

Figure 1: Fibrous hyperplasia associated with an ill-fitting prosthetic margin

❖ ***Floating ridges*** (30, 35)

This is the result of a lack of synchronization between bone resorption and fibromucosal reduction (Figure 2).

Floating ridges cause significant prosthetic instability. They limit the transmission of occlusal forces to the underlying bone. Surgical removal is necessary when they are large and fibrous without inflammatory components and are resistant to tissue conditioning.

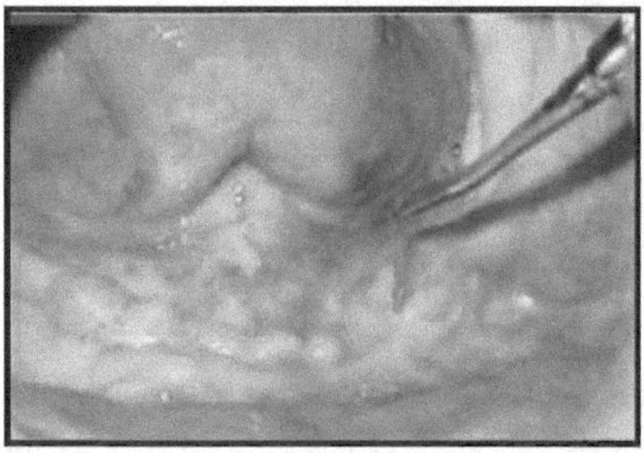

Figure 2: Fibromucosa detached from the deep plane

❖ ***Frenula and bridles close to the crest:*** (35, 43)

These cause prosthetic instability and prevent the formation of a proper peripheral seal. They must be surgically removed before the prosthesis is fabricated.

❖ ***Deepening of the oral vestibule:*** *(26)*

Modification of the position of the muscle insertions. Vestibuloplasty allows the height of the residual ridges to be increased.

1.1.2. At the bone level [67,37,26,73]

❖ ***Bone hypertrophy*** (Figure 3)*:*

Significant bone hypertrophy requires surgical intervention. These anatomical obstacles can interfere with the stability of prostheses, the extent of the bases, occlusion, and aesthetics. Even in the absence of insertion problems, these bone ridges always cause pain due to prosthetic compression (67, 37).

It can be generalized or localized. Exostosis is localized hypertrophy of the cortical bone. In the mandible, it is called mandibular torus and is most often located lingually. Treatment must take into account the etiology to prevent recurrence after surgical removal (67).

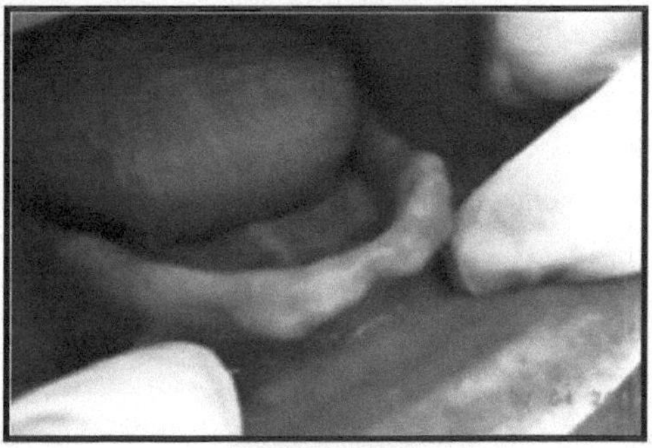

Figure 3: Bone balcony in the mandible

❖ ***Shape abnormalities:*** examples include (26, 73):

A knife-edge ridge, which causes irritation of the future prosthesis. Irregularities in the ridge resulting from poorly performed extractions.

❖ ***Hypertrophic mental spines (26):***

Following advanced resorption of the mandible, the upper mental spines are extremely prominent ( ). If the activity of the genioglossus muscle displaces the prosthesis, it would be necessary to remove the mental spine and detach this muscle.

1.2. Requirements(37,38,73,67)

The procedure must be:

- Preceded by a thorough general examination to identify any pathological processes that could potentially interfere with the desired outcome.
- A pre-surgical examination is essential.

- The clinical examination includes an exobuccal examination and an endobuccal examination. The examination of the bone tissue at the mandibular level allows the morphology of the residual crest, the position of the internal and external oblique lines, and the position and morphology of the mental spines and mandibular tori to be noted. The examination of the oral mucosa allows the condition of the mucosa covering the crest and the retromolar trigones to be determined, the position of the lingual frenulum and the anterior lip frenulum to be noted, and the extent and quality of the tissue to be removed to be assessed.
- Radiological assessment: A panoramic X-ray is always taken, and retroalveolar X-rays or a CT scan may be performed if necessary.
- Study of casts: The study model ensures accurate examination of the shape of the bone ridges.

Mounting the models on an articulator allows for evaluation of the available prosthetic space, simulation of the surgery, and fabrication of the surgical guide.

The surgical guide is a transparent resin plate prepared in advance in the laboratory on the corrected model.

- Justified
- Tissue-friendly, as all irregularities and non-painful reliefs are preserved. These will provide additional support for complete mandibular prostheses.
- Performed under anesthesia
- Followed by tissue conditioning and rigorous healing control .
- Completed with non-compressive sutures. In the mandible, it is recommended to suture without applying strong traction in order to preserve the vestibular height as much as possible.
- Post-operative medication will always be prescribed.

2. al tissue conditioning

In cases of complete mandibular edentulism, especially when long-standing, even a rigorously taken impression will only result in a prosthetic base of reduced size, incapable of ensuring the preservation of tissue integrity and the stability necessary for the restoration of various oral functions (28).

For better stability in the mandible, it is essential to increase the prosthetic support surface. Although time-consuming, tissue conditioning techniques result in considerable gains in stability and optimize the therapeutic outcome (28).

She uses delayed-setting resins and prostheses to support these materials (65).

According to Lejoyeux (52), "Conditioning refers to all the preparations and treatments designed to place the oral tissues in ideal conditions to receive a prosthesis and adapt perfectly to it."

It is particularly indicated in the presence of damaged fibromucosa that cannot fulfill its role of preserving bone tissue. Thus, tissue conditioning restores a clinically healthy appearance and normal depressibility of the mucosa.

In cases where the space reserved for the prosthesis is reduced, MECT is of major interest in restoring biofunctional space.

Similarly, following surgery, MECT promotes accelerated healing and shock absorption (65, 18, 28).

In the mandible, the support surface consists of a bone structure that is reduced in shape and volume. Generally, the space reserved for the prosthesis is invaded by paraprosthetic organs . In addition, muscle contractures are responsible for raising the reflection lines of the mucosa. This situation is common in patients with long-standing uncompensated edentulism or an old, defective prosthesis that is too small (28, 51).

According to J. Lejoyeux (54), it is essential to enlarge an extremely reduced prosthetic space before any definitive fitting. By conditioning the tissue, the prosthetic volume is gradually increased by successive applications of MECT material during the sessions.

MECT materials are delayed-setting resins, defined as plastic or elastic materials applied temporarily to the intralabial, marginal, or extralabial surfaces of a prosthesis to allow the tissues in contact with them to regain histological, anatomical, and physiological characteristics as close to normal as possible (42, 51).

Tissue conditioners are available in powder and liquid form. The powder is a polyethyl methacrylate (PEMA) or a copolymer, polyethyl and methyl methacrylate. The liquid is ethanol with aromatic esters that act as a plasticizer (most often dibutyl phthalate) (65, 30).

Several products are available on the market (Coe Comfort by Coe, Fitt by Kerr, Hydrocast by Kay See Dental MFG, Viscogel by De Trey).

Overall, an ideal tissue conditioning material should have (73):

- High initial flow to gently mold to the mucous tissues.
- Flexibility allowing the material to deform under stress.
- Elasticity to cushion masticatory forces and restore the initial shape once the force is removed.

As part of the optimization of complete mandibular prostheses, our objectives were (18, 65, 28, 73):

- An increase in the extent of the mandibular support surface by improving the shape, volume, and degree of depressibility of the mucosal reflection lines.
- Restoring the biofunctional space to an optimal volume, allowing the paraprosthetic organs to participate in the stabilization of the prosthesis in an optimal manner. The biofunctional space is the area in which the prosthesis must fit harmoniously without interfering with the surrounding muscles. The massaging action at the mucosal reflection line allows infiltrates to be eliminated. During muscle contraction, the conditioning resin placed at the edges ensures that the surrounding muscles relax. This relaxation allows the prosthetic base to extend and the prosthetic corridor to increase.
- Achieve better prosthetic balance thanks to an extension of the support surface, which improves retention and prosthetic stability.
- Better distribution of the occlusal load.

- Better psychological and physical integration of the new prosthesis. In fact, the paraprosthetic organs are accustomed to the absence of a prosthesis or to the reduced volume of the existing bases, which means that new prostheses will naturally feel unfamiliar at first.

To ensure the conditioning effect of the material, it is recommended to change the material every 3 to 4 days; a slower response is observed when the technique is used every 10 days (79).

During the tissue conditioning phase, the patient should be given the following advice (42):

- Do not eat foods that leave grains (raspberries, figs, strawberries, etc.);
- The device should be cleaned by rinsing it under water, without brushing.
- Do not place the prosthesis on paper such as Kleenex;
- Do not use hygiene products, most of which destroy retard resins.

Table I: Incompatibilities between certain resin and cleaning product combinations

<table>
<tr><th>Résine retard</th><th>Agents chimiques</th><th>Nom commercial</th></tr>
<tr><td>FITT®</td><td>Peroxydes</td><td>Steradent®</td></tr>
<tr><td>Soft-Liner®</td><td>Enzymes</td><td rowspan="3">Corega-Tabs®
Polydent®</td></tr>
<tr><td>Hydro-Cast®</td><td>Enzymes + Peroxydes</td></tr>
<tr><td>Visco-Gel®</td><td>Enzymes + Peroxydes</td></tr>
</table>

The surface of the resin can be coated with Microseal® (KAY See dental) or J-305 monopoly syrup (Factor II, Inc., Lakeside AZ). This coating is then polymerized using a simple lamp. These products help maintain the elastic qualities of the resins by preventing exchanges (79).

3. Piezography

After tooth loss, and to simulate natural conditions, artificial teeth must be fitted in harmony with the surrounding muscles.

In 1728, Fauchard, the father of modern dental surgery, said: "We must take into account the shape and contour of the external and internal surfaces of prostheses to avoid interfering with the functions of the tongue and cheeks" (53).

The more advanced the resorption of the mandibular arch, the more prosthetic retention and stability depend on the correct position of the teeth and stabilizing polished surfaces (72).

Klein (47) developed an impression technique called piezography in 1970. According to him, "Piezography is the molding of a plastic mass by intrinsic pressures generated by the peri-prosthetic muscle masses." Piezography is an interesting alternative, especially for patients who cannot undergo implant treatment. It results in complete mandibular prostheses that integrate perfectly with the functional muscle system linking anatomy and physiology, adapting form to function (72).

Improving the stability of mandibular prostheses using piezography involves exploiting the neutral space. This is the area where muscle contraction will not dislodge the prosthesis. At this level, the forces generated by the tongue pressing outward are neutralized by the forces of the buccinator-labial strap, which are applied inward (63).

With traditional impression techniques, the prosthetic support surface is recorded. With the piezographic concept, the impression records an additional dimension: a volume called the prosthetic space (19). According to Klein (47) "The available prosthetic space is neither a neutral zone nor a passive space; it is the edentulous space where the resultant horizontal forces developed by the tongue and the buccinator-labial strap must not exceed the overall retention of the prosthesis." The functions required for this prosthetic corridor molding are most often phonation and swallowing.

The use of piezographic recording techniques aims (88, 72) to:

- Better stabilization of the prosthesis:

The piezographic prosthesis is located in the prosthetic corridor. This means that contraction of the peripheral muscles presses the prosthesis against the support surface. The presence of stabilizing polished surfaces allows for functional activity in harmony with the patient's anatomy and function, resulting in better prosthetic integration.

- Greater freedom in everyday functional activities (chewing, speaking, swallowing) allows for better psychological integration of the prosthesis.
- Aesthetic improvement thanks to better facial support.
- Better prosthetic integration:

Mersel (57) explains that most mandibular prostheses made using "traditional" techniques are perceived as foreign bodies in the oral cavity and are therefore poorly integrated by patients. This is due to the absence or lack of adaptation of the prosthetic extrados to the paraprosthetic organs. In contrast, in the piezographic concept, the prosthesis is fully in line with the patient's anatomy and function and is better integrated.

- Easy prosthetic hygiene: A prosthesis made using the piezographic technique ensures close contact between the mucous membranes of the tongue, cheeks, and lips with the prosthesis's extrados, which limits stagnation and retention of food debris.

cheeks, and lips with the prosthesis's extrados, which limits stagnation and retention of food debris.

3.1. Illustration clinical

Case presentation: clinical

A 49-year-old diabetic patient presented to the removable partial denture department for prosthetic rehabilitation of his edentulous arch.

Clinical examination revealed Kennedy Applegate Class I edentulism in the maxilla and total edentulism in the mandible with Sangiolo Class IV negative ridges (Figure 11).

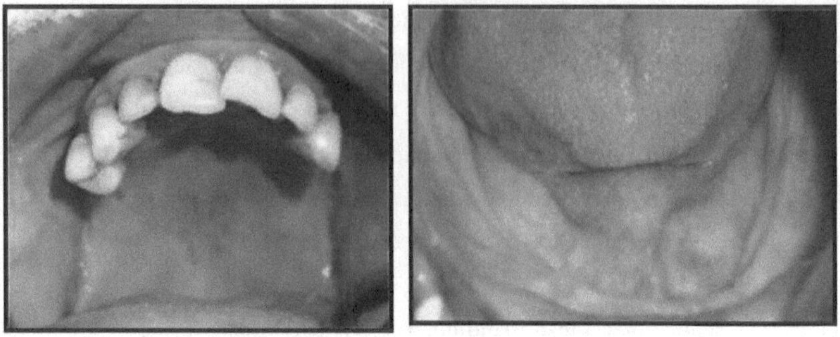

Figure 11: Maxillary and mandibular arches at consultation

cision

Following the clinical examination, we decided to fabricate a complete denture for the mandible and a removable partial denture made of resin for the maxilla.
Given the morphological deficits of the mandibular ridge, recording the prosthetic corridor seemed necessary in order to optimize the stability of the future prosthesis.

-prosthetic steps

❖ ***Piezographic impression:***

In piezography, the pre-impression described by P. Klein allowed phonetic tests to be carried out at this stage. This technique was performed without an impression tray. The material used was a polysulfide of the Surflex® Regular type.

To ensure sufficient rigidity for this impression without an impression tray, metal wire (15/10 mm) adapted to the relief of the ridge should be used, coated with an adhesive suitable for the impression material used, and would act as reinforcement (Figure 12).
First, the patient was asked to pronounce the following phonemes: "SIS" six times and "SO" once, to model the buccinator region. Next, to sculpt the anterior region of the mandible, the phonemes "TE," "DE," "SE," "ME," and "PE" were used (Figure 14).
The sequence was repeated until the material was taken. A first impression was obtained, called a pre-impression (Figure 15).
This impression was then re-margined with the same material until the prosthetic

volume was deemed satisfactory. The impression was then relined with a light polysulfide. This resulted in the final impression (Figure 16).

This impression was boxed and then cast (Figure 17).

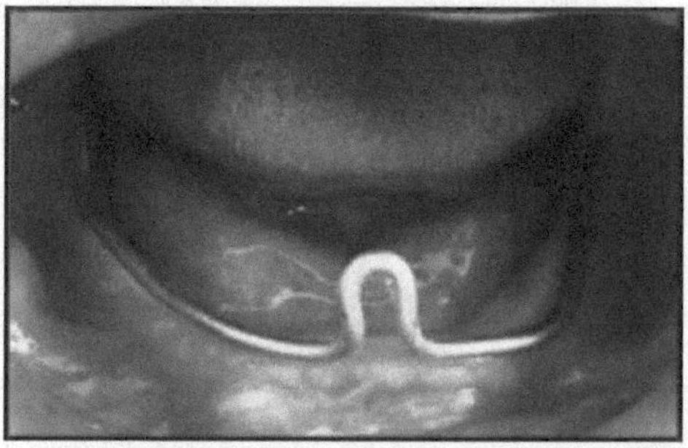

Figure 12: A reinforcement wire adapted to the morphology of the arch

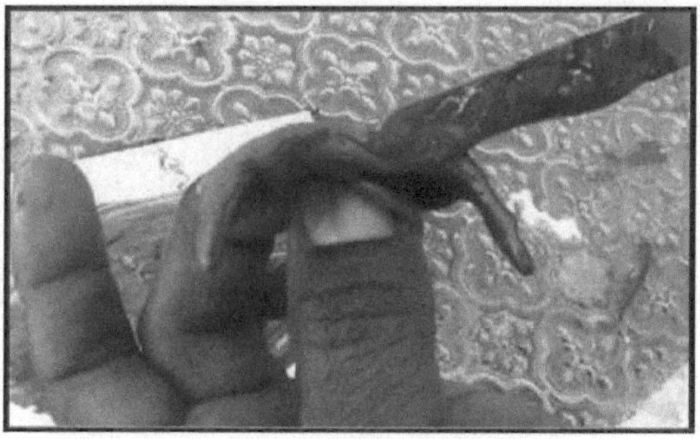

Figure 13: The wire is coated with impression material

Figure 14: The phonemes corresponding to each sector

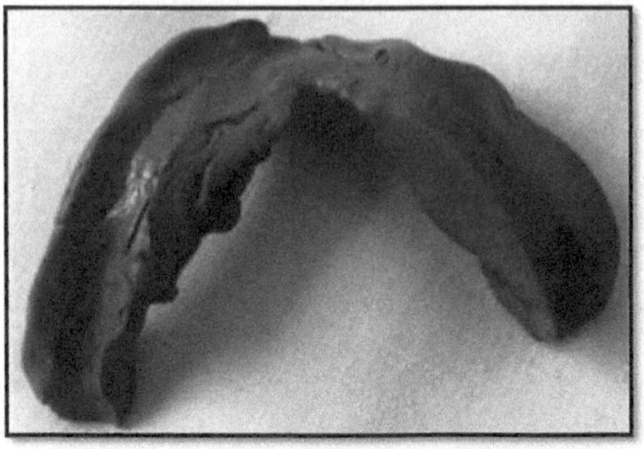

Figure 15: A pre-impression

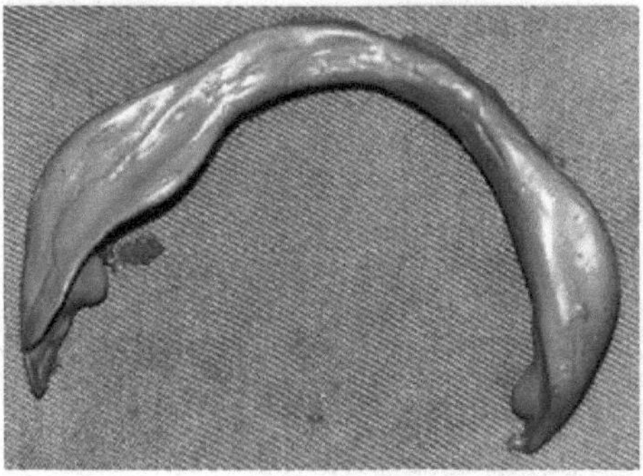

Figure 16: Final impression

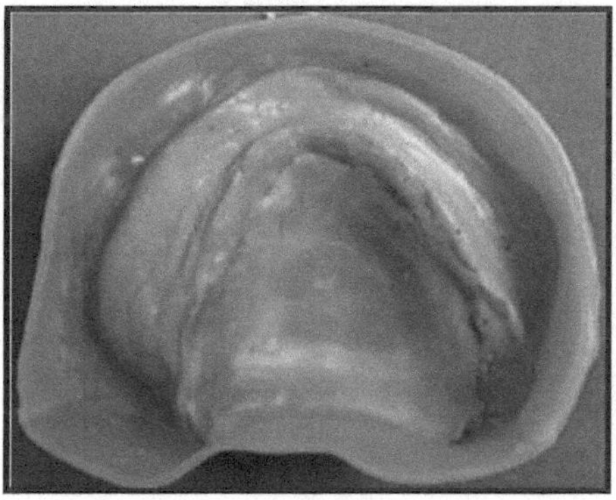

Figure 17: Boxed piezographic impression

❖ ***Construction of a rigid base:***

On the model obtained from the preliminary piezographic impression (Figure 18), a rigid base was constructed using 2 mm thick self-curing resin. It had to be stable in the mouth and cover the entire mandibular prosthetic support surface. This base was topped with a knife-edge ridge (also called a Brill ridge), perfectly centered on the arch. This ridge served as a support for the piezographic recording, which was made using a plastic material deposited on the extrados (Figure 19).

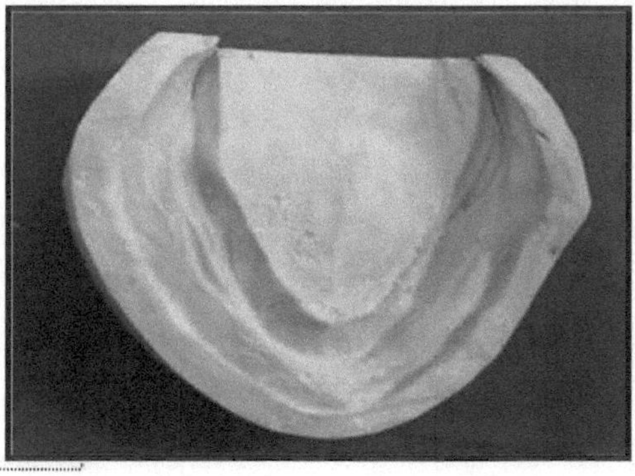

Figure 18: Model from the piezographic impression

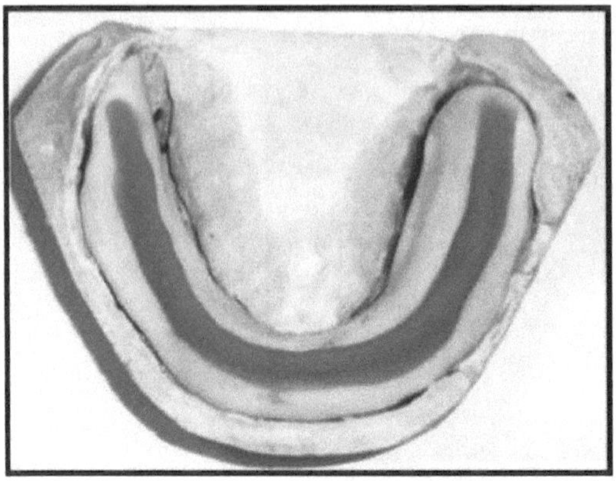

Figure 19: Self-polymerizing resin model with a knife-edge ridge

❖ ***Piezographic recording:***

The material used was a high-viscosity silicone. The mixture was placed along the model and the blade of the knife. The whole thing was inserted into the mouth.

The phonemes chosen for the modeling had to engage both sets of opposing muscles, the tongue and the buccinator-labial muscles.

The activation of the modeling during phonation was as before:

"SIS" repeated six times and "SO" once, then "TE" "DE" "SE" "ME" and "PE".

the recording the piezographic called "piezogram" (Figure 20).

It is important to note that many authors and practitioners prefer to take the secondary impression before the piezography. After checking the model, fitted with a Brill blade, the secondary impression is recorded in the usual way with a fluid silicone. Then, in the same session, piezography is performed on the Brill plate. Alternatively, the secondary impression can be taken after the piezographic recording (19).

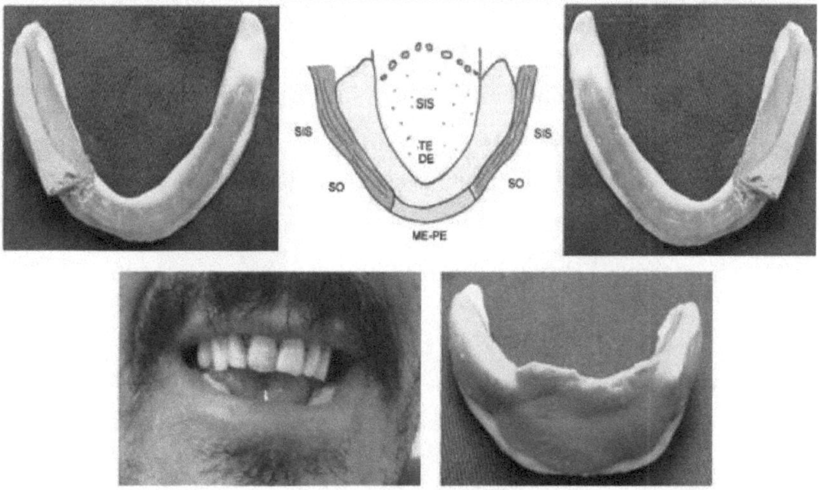

Figure 20: Obtaining the piezogram after piezographic recording using Klein's phonetic technique

❖ ***Locating the occlusal plane***

The occlusal plane was identified on the vestibular and lingual surfaces of the piezographic recording and anything protruding was cut away with a scalpel blade (Figure 21).

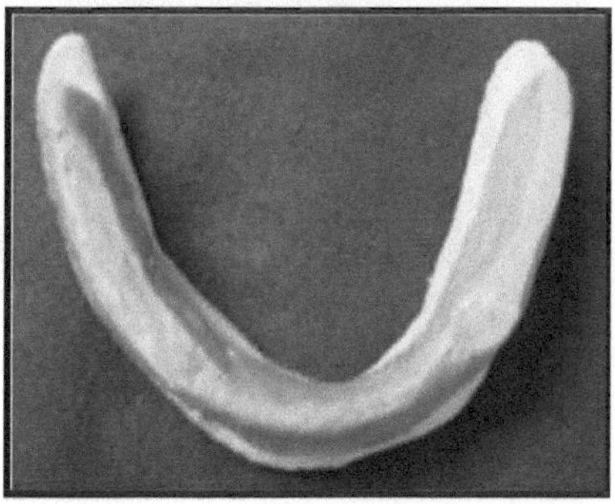

Figure 21: Occlusal plane corrected on the piezogram

The occlusal plane is determined by the muscles and is located mainly in the posterior regions of the model (72):

- Vestibular: it is located at the bottom of the grooves traced by the horizontal fibers of the buccinator muscles.
- Lingual: it corresponds to the smooth mucosal-papillary mucosal junction lines on the lateral surfaces of the tongue at rest.
- Anteriorly: according to aesthetic and phonetic rules.

❖ ***Laboratory stages:***

The piezogram was repositioned on the model created from the piezographic impression. Two vestibular and lingual keys were made from plaster around the model and the piezogram. The keys allowed both the lingual template and the position of the occlusal plane to be recorded (Figure 22).

The empty space between the two keys, once detached from the piezogram and repositioned on the mold, will give an accurate representation of the prosthetic corridor.

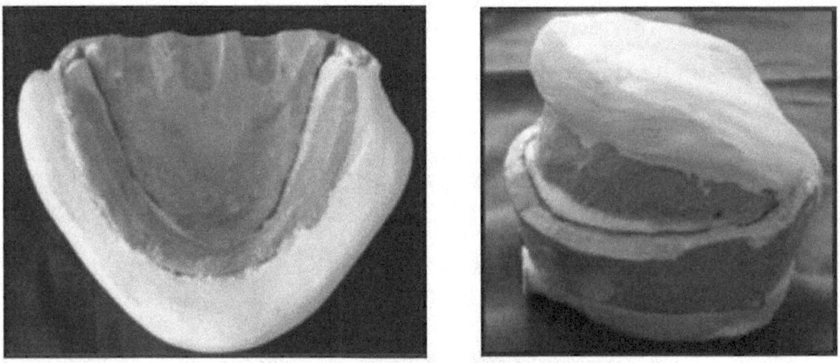

Figure 22: The two plaster vestibular and lingual keys

❖ ***Mounting the impressions on the articulator:***

To mount the upper model, resulting from a conventional impression, on a semi-adaptable articulator. Three data points were recorded in the dental office:

- The location of the maxilla in relation to the base of the skull and the hinge axis, recorded by the facebow.
- The vertical dimension of occlusion, determined in the conventional manner.
- As the occlusal plane is given by the piezographic mandibular model, only the rim of the upper model would be modified during the DVO assessment.

❖ ***Tooth mounting:***

The teeth were mounted in accordance with the morphology of the piezographic model, with the upper surface defining the position of the incisal edges and occlusal surfaces of the cuspid teeth, and the vestibular surface corresponding to the vestibular envelope of the artificial teeth (Figures 23 and 24).

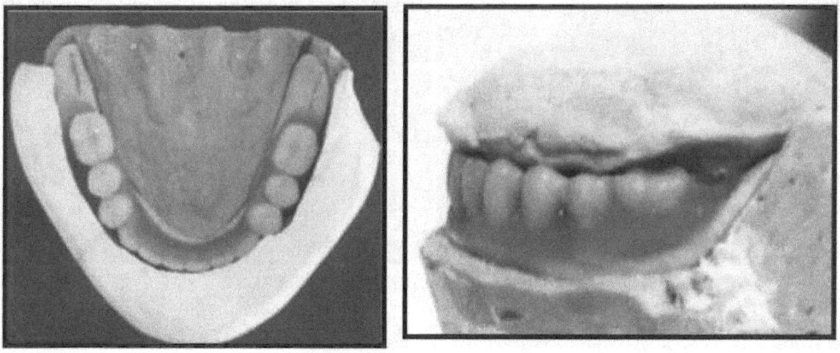

Figure 23: Mounting of teeth in accordance with the keys

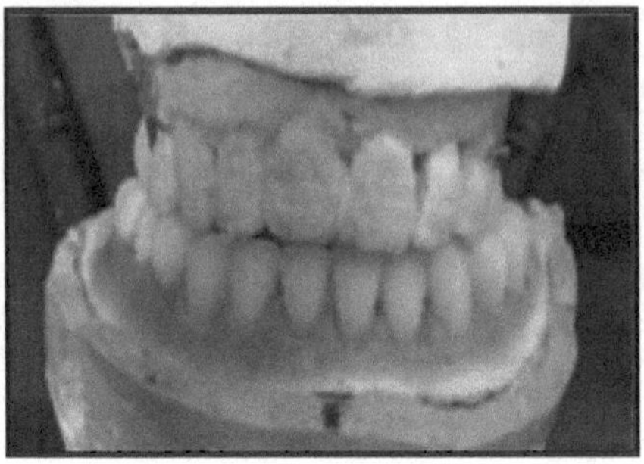

Figure 24: Mounting of teeth on articulator

- ❖ ***Wax try-in*** (Figure 25)

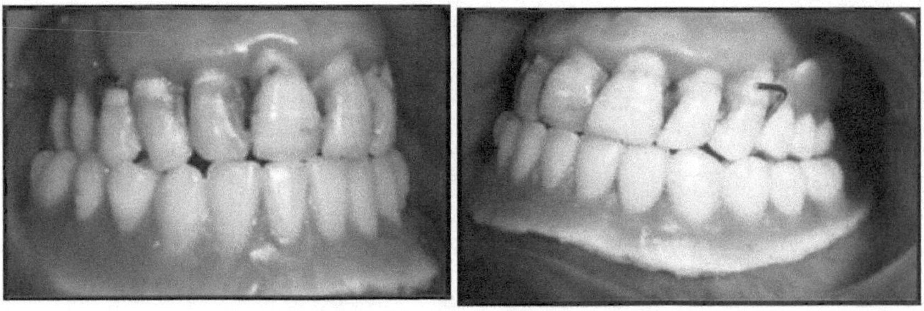

Figure 25: Trying out the teeth assembly in the mouth

- ❖ ***Placement in the mouth*** (Figure 26)

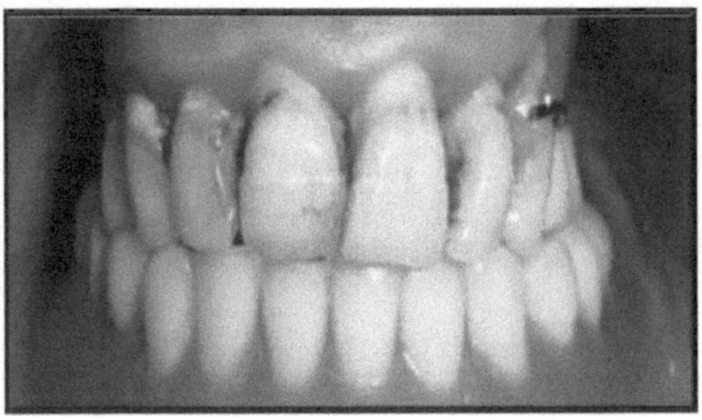

Figure 26: Fitting in the mouth

Discussion

The success of a mandibular PAC is inherent to respect for oral physiology. The assembly of the prosthetic teeth and the sculpting of the stabilizing polished surfaces must be done in harmony with muscle function. Piezography therefore contributes to therapeutic success.

Several studies have shown that piezographic prostheses are more stable than conventional prostheses during function. Comfort is also increased, and there are few post-treatment problems.

The most commonly used techniques for piezographic recording are phonation and swallowing. Other techniques have been reported in the literature, such as the water sip technique, lip pursing, functional exercises of the oral musculature, and whistling (63, 72).

In this clinical case, the practitioner used phonation as a vector for piezographic modeling. Several arguments support this technique (72, 10, 29):

- Phonation is the oral function least affected by the loss of dental and periodontal organs.
- It is considered the most developed oral function.
- Phonation, mastication, and swallowing use the same muscle effectors. However, phonation is the simplest way to energize the walls of the prosthetic space.
- It has the most permanent destabilizing muscle action. In fact, it is the source of horizontal forces that destabilize the mandibular prosthesis.
- Phonation takes place in an open cavity without interocclusal contact, which allows the recording material to escape from the oral cavity, unlike other oral functions.

Makzoumé (55) conducted a study to compare the two piezographic impression techniques: phonation and swallowing. He found that the location of the neutral zone is different for these two techniques.

The prosthetic corridor obtained using the swallowing technique is wider. However, the piezographic recording modeled by phonation is narrower only posteriorly;

anteriorly, this space is similar with both techniques.

The centrifugal action of the tongue explains this difference. The tongue pushes the recording material towards the vestibule, which is less affected by the buccinator muscles and has a weaker action during swallowing (55, 16).

The 2015 study by Nabid and Lamrous (50) demonstrated that elderly patients prefer total dentures obtained through swallowing. In fact, chewing efficiency depends on the surface area and number of occlusal contacts. Therefore, it increases with the occlusal surface area in the case of swallowing registration.

In this clinical case, the "sectoral phonetic technique" was used. During this technique, the piezographic impression is taken gradually. The impression is modeled starting with the right lateral segment, then the left, and finally the anterior segment (55).

Using the same modeling vector, phonation, it appears that the overall recording is preferred to a sectoral recording, since the vestibular and lingual volumes of the model are sculpted in their entirety (10).

A sequence of phonemes is chosen for modeling the piezographic material in the mouth. The patient is asked to read a sequence of words on a sheet held at eye level. The sequence is repeated until the material is taken (72, 29).

- For the buccinator region, the phonemes are "SIS" repeated six times, allowing the tongue to expand and the buccinator to activate, and "SO" once, causing the tongue to expand, the orbicularis to contract, and the modiolus to activate.
- For the front part of the lower jaw: the pronunciation of "TE" and "DE" ensures a centrifugal action of the tongue. The emission of "SE," "ME," and "PE" causes a centripetal action of the lips to shape the anterior external region;
- The final impression of the material is taken when the oral cavity is at rest, to record the position of muscular balance.

Depending on the patient's muscle tone, the modeling effectiveness is modified. It increases by replacing "E" with "I" or "O." Also, "ME" provides less vigorous modeling than "PE" (66).

Other authors recommend reading an interesting topic aloud and quickly. This method requires greater muscle activity, increases saliva secretion and swallowing. This will reduce the patient's attention to the occlusal ridges and the recording of muscle movements will be more natural (10, 63).

The piezography technique does have some limitations (72):

- Piezography guarantees the integration of the prosthesis into the existing anatomical and physiological context. However, it does not remove wrinkles or restore a youthful profile.
- The production time is longer than for conventional prostheses, with several difficulties in production.

- The prosthetic corridor may be very small, requiring a reduction in the vestibulo-lingual diameter of the teeth.

In 2012, Rehmann et al. (69) proposed a modified piezographic technique. This technique involved taking two alginate impressions, one of the maxilla and one of the mandible. A base plate with a wax occlusal rim was fabricated on the mandibular model obtained from the impression. The practitioner recorded the occlusion and mounted the two models on an articulator.

Next, a base plate with posterior occlusal ridges made of acrylic resin was fabricated for occlusal support (Figure 27). A cushion-type prosthetic adhesive was plasticized with hot water and applied to both
superior and inferior surfaces of the base plate created (Figure 28) (69).

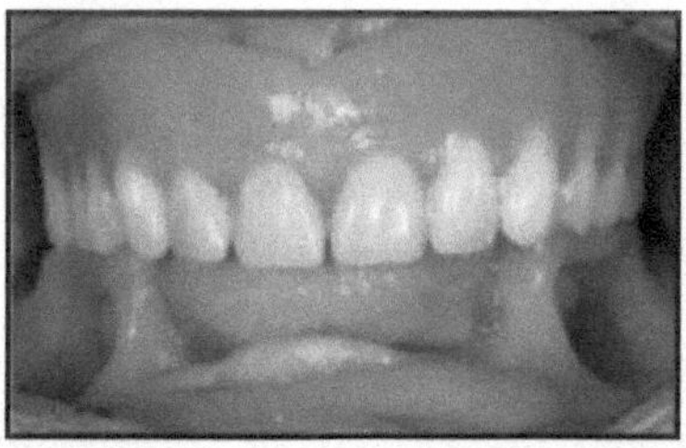

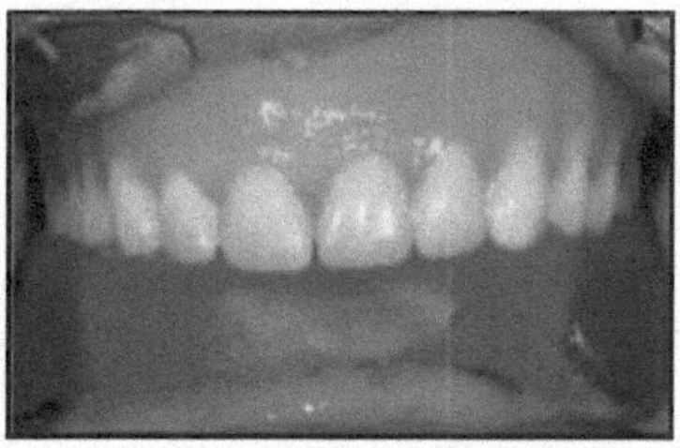

Figure 27: Base plate with posterior acrylic resin ridges, which help to fix the vertical dimension of occlusion.	Adhesive pad applied to the base plate

The patient was asked to wear the base as much as possible for two days to record the neutral zone. The base should be carefully removed and cleaned by rinsing under tap water only.

After two days, the practitioner materialized the peripheral joint with medium or low viscosity silicone. The base plate was transferred to a trial acrylic resin denture using the fluid resin technique. This denture was given back to the patient for a trial period. Then, if the patient was satisfied with the denture, silicone keys were made to mold the occlusal ridges. The teeth were mounted in accordance with these keys (69).

Rehmann P et al. (68) conducted a study to evaluate the improvement in the stability of complete mandibular dentures using a modified piezographic impression technique. They noted a significant improvement in oral health-related quality of life in the majority of patients. A high percentage of patients reported an improvement in the overall stability of the prosthesis during chewing (85.7%) and, to a lesser extent, during phonation (66.7%). However, no significant change in masticatory function was observed.

This technique is recommended mainly in cases of compromised ridges and when implant treatment is contraindicated. However, it cannot be recommended for routine clinical use due to its complexity. It also requires detailed and demanding instructions for both the patient and the prosthetist.

4. ly stabilizing polished surfaces

Stabilizing polished surfaces are areas on the prosthetic extrados that allow the paraprosthetic musculature to participate in balancing the prosthesis and facilitating food evacuation.

As early as 1933, Fish was interested in the importance of the shape and polish of stabilizing polished surfaces. He proposed semi-empirical stabilizing profiles. With further developments, it was recommended that these surfaces be recorded through muscle activity (66).

Stabilizing polished surfaces are obtained either by sculpting the wax or using specific piezographic impression techniques (35).

4.1. Roles of prosthetic extrados [66,35,36]

- Optimization of facial aesthetics: The shape and volume of prosthetic extrados, combined with correct tooth mounting, ensure support for paraprosthetic organs (66).
- Improved physical retention: Physical retention is influenced by the extent of the contact surface between the prosthesis and the surrounding tissues. The presence of stabilizing polished surfaces increases contact between the prosthesis, the salivary film, and the paraprosthetic organs.
- Achieving muscle retention: When the prosthetic extrados

divergent planes toward the support surface, even at rest, the paraprosthetic muscles (cheeks, lips, and tongue) will press the prostheses against the osteomucosal support tissues (Figure 29).

During function, it appears that contraction of the stabilizing muscles, such as the buccinators and orbicularis oris, improves retention.

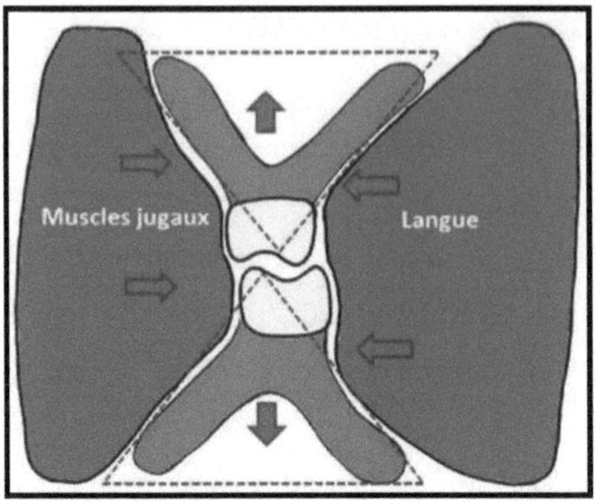

Figure 29: Action of the buccal muscles and tongue on their inclined prosthetic extrados

- Better stabilization of the prosthesis: Polished surfaces stabilize the prosthesis by balancing the pressure between the labial, jugal, and lingual muscle components, promoting the action of stabilizing muscles and inhibiting the action of destabilizing muscles (66, 36).
- Improvement of various oral functions such as phonation, mastication, and swallowing (66).

4.2. Indications [66]

- Lack of retention and stability of the prosthesis due to severe ridge resorption.
- The presence of destabilizing scar tissue.
- Presence of depressible tissue or floating ridges.
- Patients with specific phonetic requirements (wind instrument players, singers).
- Certain cases of maxillofacial prosthetic restoration.

•

4.3.Polished surfaces obtained by sculpting the wax

The stabilizing polished surfaces are traditionally sculpted according to certain rules. The lingual profile in the incisor-canine area has a double horizontal and vertical concavity, called the lingual cradle, which helps keep the tongue in a low position and plays a role in stabilizing the prosthesis. The rest of the lingual area should not have any undercuts (Figure 30). On the vestibular side, the profiles are designed with alternating concavities and convexities. A concavity in the incisive region ensures freedom of movement of the orbicularis oris muscle and restores harmony to the lips through the design of the labio-mental sulcus. A concavity at the premolars allows for the dynamics of the muscular junction of the modiolus (Figure 31) (36).

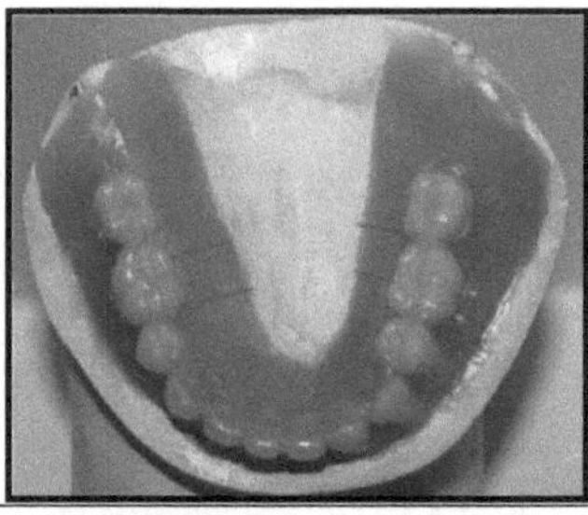

Figure 30: Mandibular prosthesis with inclined planes (in red) and a lingual cradle (in blue) (35)

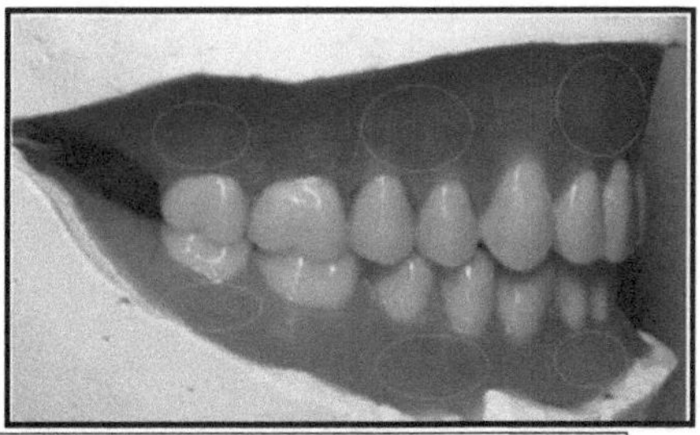

Figure 31: Lateral vestibular extrados (35)

Table II: Two methods of sculpting polished surfaces according to RIGNON-BRET C and HÜE O. (70, 35, 44, 66)

	RIGNON-BRET C	HUE O.
Vestibular level		
Incisal area	A concavity for the orbicularis oris muscle.	Concavity
The canine region	A slight convexity limiting the canine bump.	Convexity (between canine and 1st premolar)
The premolar region	A concavity	Premolar (betw The distal of th 1e concavity een face mesial e 2e premolar) and opposit the e
The region molar, opposite Fish's pockets.	A convexity	Convexity (from the second premolar to the central part of the second molar)
The posterior area of the Fish pocket	A slight concavity to allow free movement of the masseter	Distal concavity (for the buccinator and masseter)
At the lingual level		
At the of the sublingual region	A double concavity in the anteroposterior and mesiodistal direction, known as the lingual cradle	Concavity between the submaxillary and sublingual regions: more pronounced concavity
At the posterior level	No undercuts to prevent the prosthesis from being lifted by the tongue.	Concavity
Posterior posterior of lingual flaps	Follows the profile of the bearing surfaces	

4.4. The polished surfaces obtained by dynamic recording (62,66,14,76)

The masseteric strap can be recorded either immediately after the secondary impression or after recording the intermaxillary relationships. This impression allows the volume and functional incidence of the active false gingiva to be validated and corrected (62).

4.4.1. Materials used (66)

Plastic waxes at mouth temperature, slow-setting resins or elastomers are generally used on the extrados of the individual impression tray (PEI) or wax model to take an impression of the paraprosthetic tissues.

4.4.2. The technique (62)

There are two stages: a clinical stage and a laboratory stage.

- ***At the dental practice:***

After the primary and secondary impressions, the practitioner records the occlusion and mounts the secondary models on an articulator.

Next, they check the action of the masseters on the occlusal base. They place their index fingers on the extrados of the mandibular base at the level of the Fish pocket and ask the patient to contract their masseters. The practitioner should feel their fingers pressing against the mandibular occlusal base. This movement is repeated until it is mastered by the patient.

Next, an adhesive is placed on the extrados of the occlusal base at the level of the Fish pockets, and the patient's gums are coated with petroleum jelly to prevent the impression material from adhering to this area. The occlusal bases are inserted into the oral cavity with the silicone interposed.

The impression material is mixed, placed in an impression syringe, and injected between the corner of the mouth and the upper surface of the mandibular base at the right and left Fish pockets (Figure 32). The patient is asked to repeat the masseter contraction movements.

This impression is surfaced again by injecting the same material but in a more fluid form. Finally, the impression is removed from the oral cavity, checked, and sent to the laboratory.

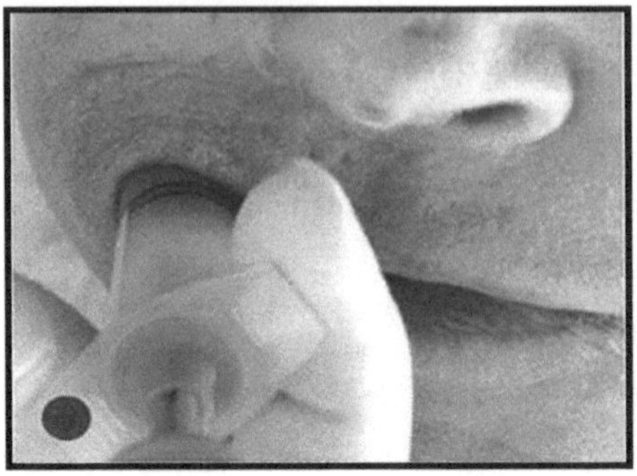

Figure 32: Recording of the prosthetic extrados

❖ ***In the laboratory:***

The prosthetist makes heavy silicone keys from the impression obtained.

The prosthetic teeth are mounted in the usual way, ensuring aesthetics and function. In the anterior region, the false gingiva is sculpted in the usual way, but in the posterior regions, the keys are used to sculpt the functional false gingiva.

When trying out the teeth on wax, the practitioner should examine the shape of the false gum.

Unfortunately, the technique described ignores the polished lingual and anterior vestibular surfaces.

Manually sculpted polished surfaces generally describe concavities along the vestibular surfaces. However, the contours resulting from the functional impression lead to generalized convexities along the vestibular surfaces of mandibular dentures.

Stromberg et al. (76) compared dentures with manually sculpted polished surfaces and those obtained by dynamic registration. They found that all patients preferred the manually sculpted dentures. It appears that the exaggerated contours of the functional prosthesis le d to a slight decrease in retention during the different degrees of mouth opening used in the study (62, 14, 76).

5. Role of occlusion in prosthetic stability

In complete dentures, occlusion describes specific criteria in static and dynamic terms.

- Static occlusion is characterized by the occlusal plane, position and orientation, as well as the correct vertical dimension of occlusion in centric relation.
- Dynamic occlusion is influenced by the morphology of artificial teeth and their assembly, which determines the occlusal pattern (39).

5.1. Occlusal concepts in complete removable prostheses

The occlusal concept is the set of rules establishing the number and location of contacts for the meshing of teeth and sliding surfaces, in the reference position and during mandibular movements (75).

5.1.1. Conventional balanced occlusion [4,20]

This pattern is defined by occlusal contacts between the mandibular buccal cusps and the maxillary central fossae on one side, and between the maxillary palatal cusps and the mandibular central fossae on the other side (Figure 35). The compensatory curves, anteroposterior and mediolateral, result in non-working lateral contacts during lateral and propulsive movements.

propulsion. This promotes stability during function.

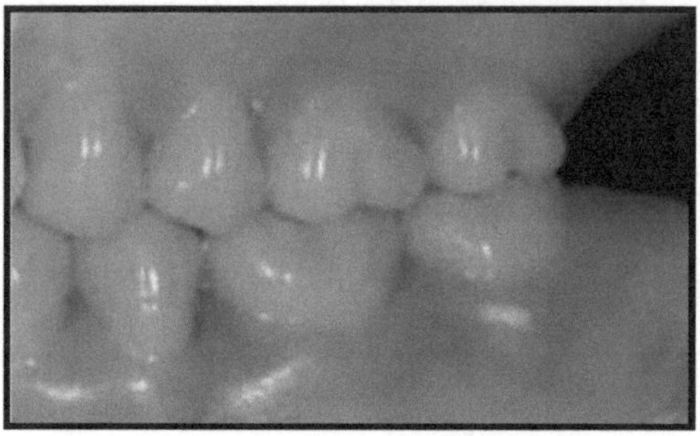

Figure 35: Balanced balanced occlusion [20]

5.1.2. [A]balanced lingualized occlusion [4,20,25,78,46]

This concept is characterized by maxillary palatal cusps in contact with the mandibular central fossae, with no contact between the mandibular vestibular cusps and the maxillary central fossae. Only the palatal cusps, on the working side and non-working side, are in contact during lateral movements (Figure 36) (4, 20).

Improved stability of the lower denture during chewing is suggested when this concept is followed (4).

Deniz and Ozken (25) compared masticatory efficiency, prosthesis performance, and patient satisfaction for two occlusal schemes, lingualized occlusion and balanced occlusion, in cases of extreme resorption. The study showed that chewing performance was better with lingualized occlusion. Retention and prosthetic stability were also improved with lingualized occlusion.

In addition, other advantages were observed when teeth were mounted according to balanced lingual occlusion: improved comfort, patient satisfaction, phonation, and aesthetics (78, 46).

Finally, this concept simplifies contact balancing. A reduced frequency of prematurity is noted compared to conventional balanced occlusion (20).

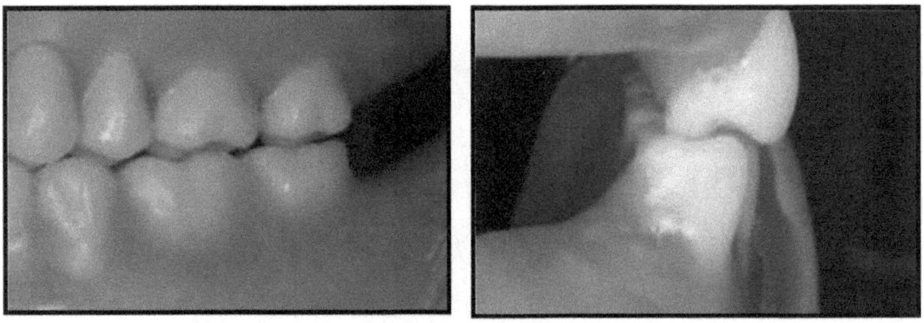

Figure 36: Lingualized balanced occlusion

5.1.3. Monoplanar occlusion [4,20]

Occlusal contacts comprise surfaces rather than points due to the use of non-anatomical posterior prosthetic teeth ( ) (Figure 37d).

This scheme is suggested in the presence of a resorbed lower ridge and skeletal bases in Class II Div 1 or Class III to reduce the resulting instability of interferences.

With monoplanar occlusion, the absence of cusps prevents contacts from being maintained during lateral movements.

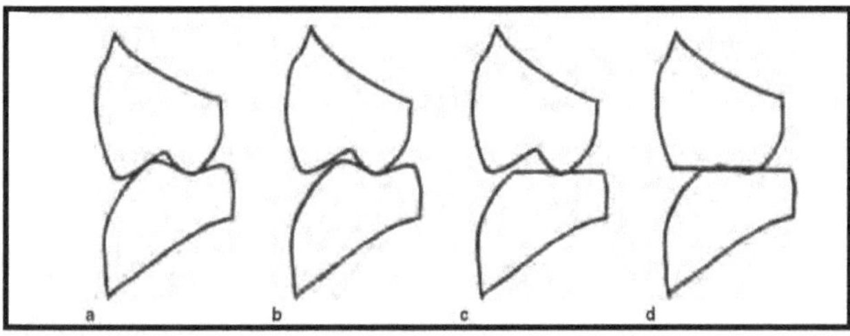

Figure 37: Modification of the morphology and arrangement of posterior teeth: (a) anatomical teeth arranged in balanced occlusion; (b) anatomical teeth arranged in lingualized balanced occlusion; (c) anatomical maxillary teeth and flat mandibular teeth arranged in lingualized balanced occlusion; (d) flat teeth arranged in monoplan occlusion [4]

6. Contribution of prosthetic adhesives

The use of prosthetic adhesives is considered a useful therapeutic adjunct to improve the retention and stability of complete dentures, particularly mandibular dentures (60). These adhesives first appeared in modern dentistry at the end of the 18th century, with their first application described in late 1913. Although followed by other patents in 1920 and 1930, it was not until 1935 that adhesives were first mentioned in the dental literature by the American Dental Association Council on Dental Materials, Instruments, and Equipment as non-medical products (60, 48). Adhesives are commercially available, non-prescription products defined as a dental supply applied to the intralabial surface of a removable prosthesis to temporarily improve the retention and stability of prostheses (59, 9).

There are two types of adhesives: "soluble" adhesives, which include creams, strips (or bands), and powders; and "insoluble" adhesives in the form of pads (48).

6.1. Composition [60,59,9]

Depending on their composition, they can be classified as natural or synthetic adhesives (60).

Adhesives consist of four product families: adhesive agents, adjuvants, coloring and flavoring substances, and various ingredients.

6.1.1. Adhesive agents [59,9]

These are mixtures of short- and long-acting synthetic polymers that hydrate and expand to fill the gaps between the prosthesis and the mucous tissues. Two types of adhesive agents are mainly used:

1. Carboxymethylcellulose (CMC) is a synthetic gel derived from cellulose, insoluble in water and providing rapid adhesive action. It forms a viscous solution when in contact with an aqueous medium, creating rapid ionic adhesion with the prosthesis and the epithelium of the oral mucosa.
2. PVM/MA salts: These take longer than CMC to hydrate and, at high concentrations, increase adhesion and viscosity. They provide prolonged adhesive action.

The ratio of CMC to PVM/MA has a significant effect on the viscosity of adhesives.

6.1.2. Adjuvant

These are composed of fatty substances (petroleum jelly, mineral oil, polyethylene oxide) that bind the various components together. Adjuvants also facilitate the application of the product (9).

6.1.3. Flavoring substances and coloring agents

They are generally derived from essential oils (mint or chamomile oil) and synthetic colorants (9).

6.1.4. Ingredients , etc.

Other ingredients may be found (9):

- Antioxidants with vitamin E action (tocopherol).
- Antimicrobial agents (sodium tetraborate, ethanol, hexachlorophene, etc.).
- "Soothing" agents with "anti-inflammatory" properties, derived from chamomile or licorice.

6.2. Criteria for an ideal adhesive [6]

According to Adisman (6), it must meet seven criteria:

1. Biocompatible, non-toxic, and non-irritating,
2. Does not promote the growth of microorganisms,
3. Neutral odor and taste,
4. Easy to apply and remove from the underside of the prosthesis,
5. Persistent adhesive potential for 12 to 16 hours,
6. Available in cream or gel form
7. Increased comfort, stability, and retention of the prosthesis.

6.3. Advantages [59,60]

The use of adhesive is associated with feelings of comfort, satisfaction, and self-confidence in social interactions. This is achieved through:

- Improved retention and stability of removable dentures.
- Reduced movement of dentures during cutting and chewing.
- A barrier role that prevents or reduces the migration of food particles under the prosthesis.

6.4. Disadvantages [60,79]

- Adhesives lead to avoidance of good clinical practices by dentists.
- For patients, adding increasing amounts of adhesive may be a solution to poorly fitting dentures rather than seeking professional care.
- The use of adhesives can mask problems with the prosthesis.
- Regular care and follow-up are necessary.

6.5. Indications and contraindications [79,9,59,6]

First and foremost, the denture used must be adequate and suitable for healthy mucous tissue. In the presence of unstable, non-retentive, or fractured dentures, or in patients unable to maintain good denture hygiene or oral hygiene, denture adhesives should be avoided.

Furthermore, the authors (9, 59, 79, 6) recommend the judicious use of these products in the following situations:

- Presence of anatomical areas with poor retention: due to the shape of the ridge and the quality of the mucous membranes.
- Psychological support for patients who find it difficult to accept new removable prostheses.
- Patients wearing immediate dentures.
- Xerostomic patients with removable prostheses.
- Patients with maxillofacial prostheses.
- In the presence of mucous membranes that are thin due to age or susceptible to irritation due to lack of lubrication: the adhesive can act as a cushion for the mucous membranes.

6.6. Use

Patients should be informed that the adhesive should be used sparingly and, if ne , that excessive application, in terms of quantity or frequency, may indicate that the dentures have become ill-fitting. They should understand that, over time and with inevitable bone resorption, their dentures will need to be readjusted or relined. It is important to note that the adhesive is not intended to replace this procedure (59).

Zinc-free adhesives are recommended. For adhesives containing zinc, consumers should follow the manufacturer's instructions for use.

The use of prosthetic adhesives over long periods without periodic check-ups by a dentist is contraindicated (59, 48).

Compliance with the rules for application, use, and removal of adhesives ensures their optimal use.

Prosthetic adhesives must be applied in accordance with certain recommendations (9):

- The underside of the denture must be cleaned and dried.
- For creams, apply three pea-sized increments of adhesive cream to the underside (Figure 38).

For powder adhesives, the intralabial surface must be moistened with water. It is recommended to sprinkle a thin layer of adhesive over the entire surface of the intralabial surface, then remove any excess.

In the case of adhesive strips, place the strip of the correct size on the underside of the prosthesis and trim off any excess with scissors.

- The prosthesis must be placed in the mouth and held firmly in place for 5 to 10 seconds.
- The patient should remove any excess material from the cheek or tongue.
- Finally, the patient is asked to bite down firmly to spread the product and remove any excess from the denture.

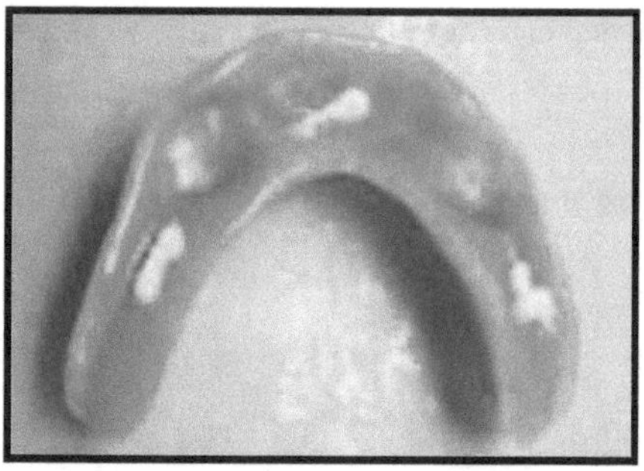

Figure 38: Application of adhesive cream to the lower denture

Thorough cleaning of adhesives is difficult and delicate, especially for elderly people or those with limited mobility (9).

It is recommended that the adhesive be removed daily. The procedure consists of four steps (9):

1. Carefully remove the dentures using only your fingers to avoid injury.
2. Brushing the oral cavity to remove any adhesive residue from the mucous membranes.
3. Brushing the dentures with a brush and a suitable cleaning agent.
4. Soak the denture in a suitable product.

6.7. Comparison of denture adhesives (60,59,48,9)

The retention time of adhesives varies between 3 and 12 hours, depending on the type. Adhesive pads remain effective after 10 hours, while adhesive creams remain active for more than 4 hours but less than 10 hours. This difference in duration of action can be explained by the solubility of cream adhesives (60).

Creams perform better than strips. The difference is due to the fact that strips do not contain long-acting synthetic polymers. (59, 60)

Adhesive pads provide the greatest increase in masticatory capacity. In fact, thanks to their varying thickness, they act as a relining material, adapting to the supporting tissues and the prosthetic intraoral surface (60, 48).

Maximum retention forces were observed with new dentures on substantial bone ridges, but the difference is greater for older dentures on weak ridges (9).

Use of tooth roots

The preservation of teeth and residual roots, with the aim of improving the retention and stability of complete mandibular prostheses, is a long-standing concept. When only tooth roots remain on the arch, it is recommended to preserve these roots and fabricate a supra-radicular prosthesis (2, 29).

1. Conditions for the use of tooth roots:

The use of these residual roots must comply with certain conditions, namely:

- The intraosseous root height must be at least half the root height (8 to 10 mm) with no root mobility before loading (5).
- An attached gingival barrier (minimum 2 mm) to ensure the longevity of the teeth.
- A root axis favorable to the preparation and reception of a mechanical system (29, 2).
- The distribution of the remaining teeth on the arch: incidentally, the presence of teeth on the same side contraindicates supra-radicular prostheses due to the risks of unilateral chewing, accentuated resorption of the edentulous hemi-arch, and rotation of the prosthesis around the remaining teeth (5, 2).

Prosthetic balance is improved when the residual roots are distributed on both sides of the arch. This means either four symmetrically distributed roots, three roots that are spaced and distributed, or two roots on either side of the median sagittal plane. Thanks to their strategic positions, the two mandibular canines are the most commonly used teeth in PACSR.

Spacing between abutments is essential for prosthesis stability, reducing the risk of periodontal damage and facilitating hygiene measures. (2, 82)

- Sufficient prosthetic space is required to accommodate the volume of the attachments (2).

2. Advantages of preserving tooth roots in the mandible:

Support and stabilization are provided entirely by the complete mandibular prosthesis, and the residual roots are used to place attachments that provide additional retention (70).

Preserving these teeth, even as roots, ensures comfort and psychological acceptance of the future complete mandibular prosthesis. Another important point is the preservation of periodontal proprioception, which ensures the maintenance of neuromuscular coordination and therefore masticatory efficiency of up to 90% (2, 29). Furthermore, this option is a simple and attractive solution that significantly reduces bone loss in the mandible (Figure 60) and maintains alveolar volume

that guarantees favorable support surfaces for suspension and stabilization (15, 2).

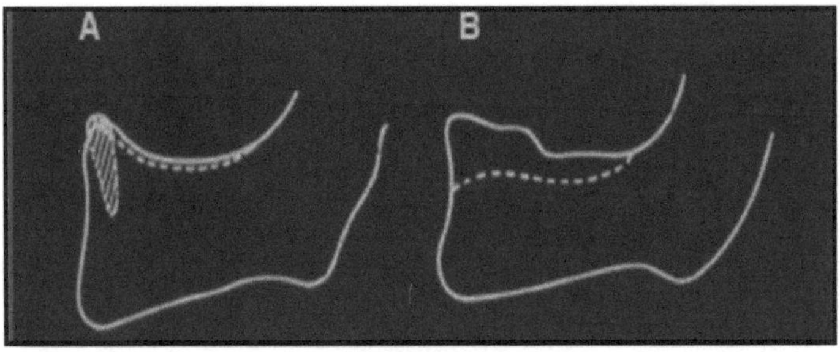

Figure 60: Comparison of bone loss in (A) a patient with a supra-radicular prosthesis and (B) a conventional complete denture 5 years after tooth extraction and prosthesis insertion of dentures (15)

3. Choice of attachment system:

Retention is increased through the use of the attachment system (2).

In fact, the choice is between two types of attachments that are frequently used: axial attachments and anchor bars.

This device must also meet certain requirements (29):

- Simple design and easy maintenance for both the practitioner and the patient.

- Sufficient retention force of 10 to 20 N.
- Reliability: wear causes a reduction in retention, which must be compensated for by activating or changing the retention rings.

A set of criteria were studied to guide our choice (70, 5, 29):

- **The shape of the crest:**

A straight anterior ridge favors the use of a connecting bar. The bar is contraindicated for a curved anterior ridge to avoid crowding in the lingual envelope and harmful biomechanical stresses on the roots. Axial attachments are indicated regardless of the shape of the anterior ridge.

- **Tooth axis:**

With the bar, parallelism of the root axes is recommended. However, the presence of non-parallel abutments is not a major contraindication; this problem can be solved by screwing a bar onto one of the abutments.

The standard ball attachment is contraindicated when the non-parallelism exceeds 10°. In this case, it can create harmful stresses on the roots and increase the need for maintenance of the attachment system.

- **The periodontal value of teeth:**

When residual canines have a CR/RR ratio of 1, the use of a bar allows for a kind of retention of the two roots. Thanks to the stabilization of the abutment teeth, this device reduces stress during movement and relieves the periodontal tissues of the abutments. It should be noted that the bar is contraindicated when the roots have very uneven periodontal values; the use of axial attachments will be safer.

- **The usable prosthetic volume in the areas concerned:**

The guide assembly allows for an accurate estimate of the usable prosthetic volume s (height, mesiodistal width, and vestibulolingual width) (Figure 61).

Due to its spacing from the edentulous ridge, the bar requires more space than the axial attachment.

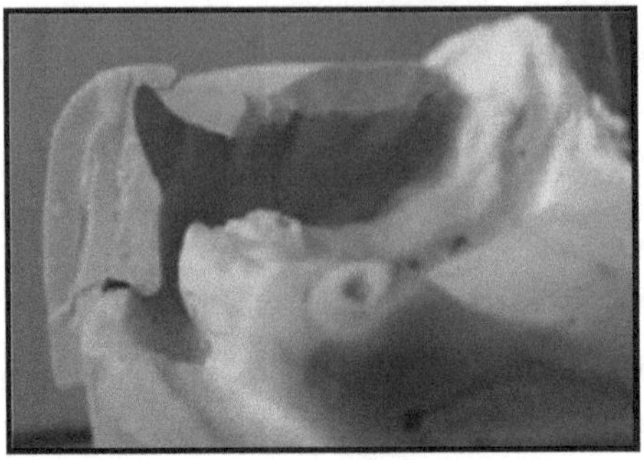

Figure 61: Evaluation of the available prosthetic space using silicone keys made on the master model

For PACSR, the difference in depressibility between the fibromucosa and the tooth roots must be taken into account when choosing an attachment. The attachment must contain axial play to ensure vertical translation and/or angular play for distal rotation (70, 12).

From a technical standpoint, the implementation of the bar is relatively difficult compared to axial attachments; however, it provides increased prosthetic stability and complete patient satisfaction (82).

Maintaining the result obtained depends on the patient maintaining impeccable oral and prosthetic hygiene. This oral hygiene is facilitated by leaving a space between the gingival flap and the bar. This space is necessary and must be sufficient to allow interdental brushes to pass through. If it is too large, it facilitates hygiene but makes it difficult to insert the prosthetic teeth and increases the risk of diapneusia in the long term, or if it is insufficient, it causes inflammation of the underlying mucosa (29).

Hue et al. (43) reported a loss of 5 to 20% of the supporting roots of PACSRs despite rigorous hygiene.

4. Clinical illustration

A 51-year-old patient presented to the removable partial denture department at the Monastir dental clinic for cosmetic and functional reasons. The patient was in good general health.

The intraoral examination revealed moderately adequate oral hygiene.

In the maxillary arch:

- The dento-periodontal factor: a defective temporary bridge was noted, with teeth 13, 12, 21, 22, and 23 as abutment teeth (Figure 39).

These teeth had a CR/RR ratio of less than 1. Tooth 22 was in root form but was well implanted in the bone.

- The osteomucosal factor: The maxillary crest was high, wide, and covered with firm, adherent fibromucosa. The right tuberosity showed undercutting due to a recent extraction.

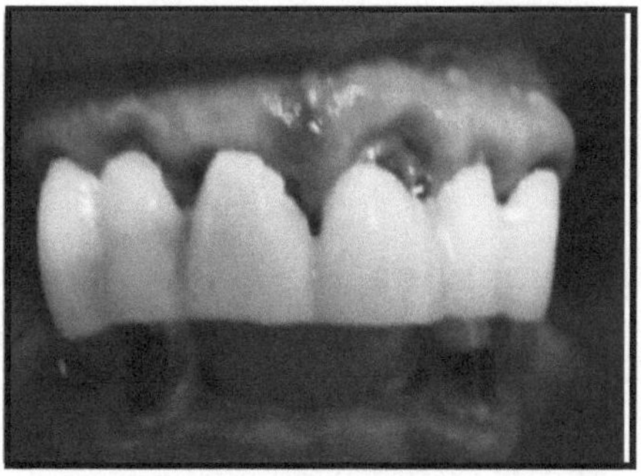

Figure 39: Defective temporary bridge

At the level of the mandibular arch:

- Dento-periodontal factor: The two canines were found to be alive but had cervical caries limited to the dentin, gingival inflammation due to tartar, and periodontal recession of 2 to 3 mm (Figure 40).

The CR/RR ratio, as shown on the retroalveolar radiographs (Figure 41), was equal to 1 and the mobility of these teeth was grade 1.

• Osteomucosal factor: The anterior mandibular edentulous ridge was straight, relatively high, and covered with adherent fibromucosa, while the ridges in the posterior sectors had a moderately favorable relief.

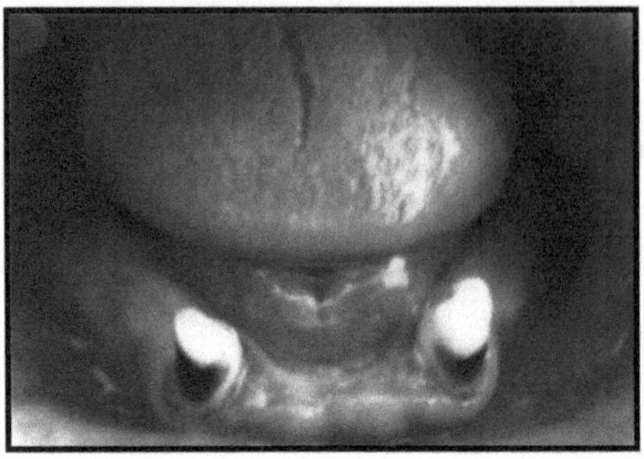

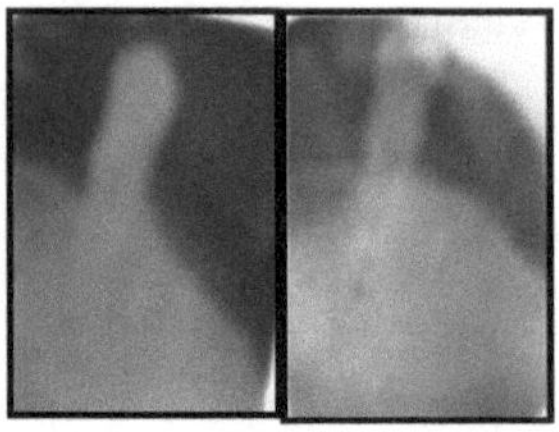

Figure 40: Subtotal mandibular edentulism	Figure 41: Retro-alveolar canines

a. -prosthetic treatments

- Motivating the patient to practice good oral hygiene
- Scaling and root planing
- Removal of defective temporary bridge.
- Treatment of cavities in the mandibular canines, followed by technical pulpectomy.

b. Prosthetic diagnosis

- Class and extent of tooth loss:
  - In the maxilla: Kennedy Applegate Class I, extensive.
  - In the mandible: Subtotal edentulism.
- Dento-periodontal factor: Favorable in the maxilla and moderately favorable in the mandible.
- Osteomucosal factor: Favorable.
- Occlusal diagnosis
  - Occlusal plane: to be restored
  - DVO: not preserved
  - PIM: absent

- HOPU sufficient
- Anterior guide: Dysfunctional.

c. Decision r prosthetic

- In the maxilla: Composite prosthesis with Preci-Vertix extracoronal attachments at 13 and 23.

- Mandible: Complete prosthesis on a connecting bar. We opted for the anchor bar rather than axial attachments due to the average periodontal value of the residual canines. The use of the bar ensures root retention and provides better retention than axial attachments.
- This decision could only be confirmed after mounting the study casts on an RC-DVO articulator and assessing the available vertical height. The position of the bar in the vertical plane also required the mounting of the mandibular prosthetic teeth.

After removing the crowns from the plaster cast, a preliminary assembly was carried out on the study cast, taking into account the aesthetic and balance requirements of the complete denture (Figure 42). Next, two silicone keys were made on this assembly (Figures 43 and 45). Once the assembly was removed, these keys made it possible to visualize the relationship between the prosthetic teeth and the root plates (Figures 44 and 46).

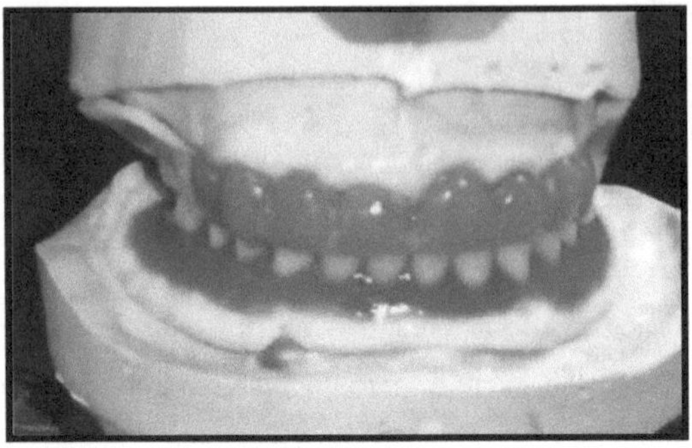

Figure 42: Director's montage

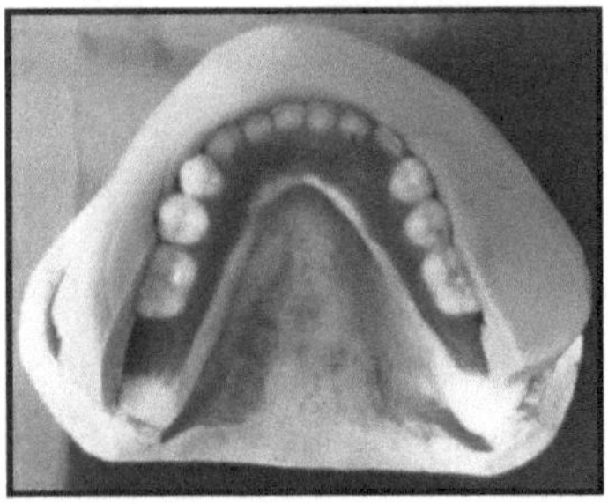

Figure 43: Vestibular situation key

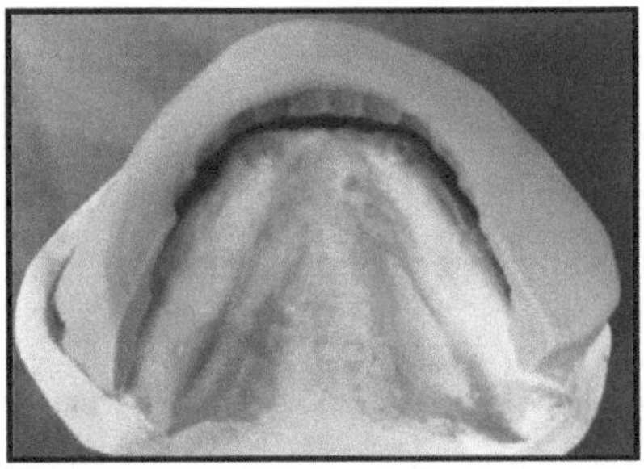

Figure 44: Visualization of space available in the vertical direction

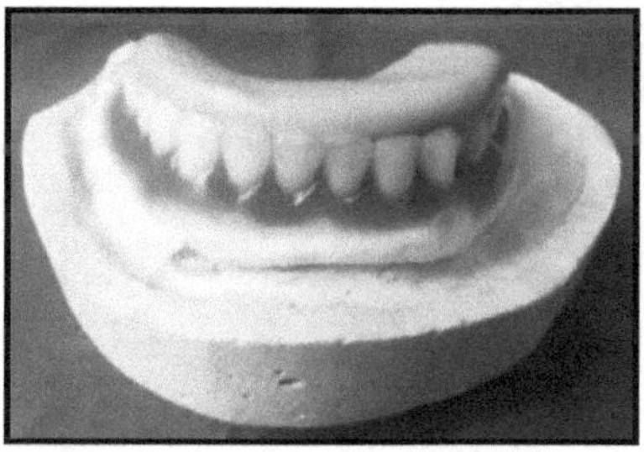

Figure 45: Lingual position key in the horizontal direction

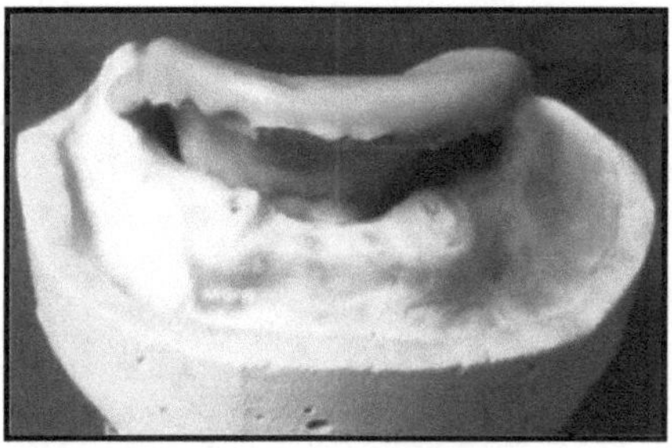

Figure 46: Visualization of available space

d. Presentation of the selected bar system: The Preci-Horix

This system includes (Figure 47):

1. A circular section bar made of calcinable resin that extends into a plate that can be adapted to the shape of the ridge.
2. A resin rider ensures the retention of the removable prosthesis.
3. A resin matrix that allows the rider to be positioned in the prosthesis after the resin has polymerized.
4. Instrument for inserting the rider.

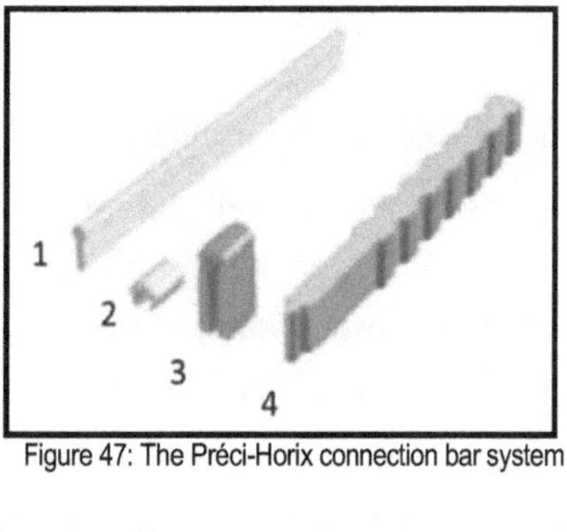

Figure 47: The Préci-Horix connection bar system

e. Sequence of steps for creating a prosthetic

Preparation of the two canines: after scaling, root planing, and endodontic treatment, the two canines were prepared in the manner of a Richmond plate (Figure 48).

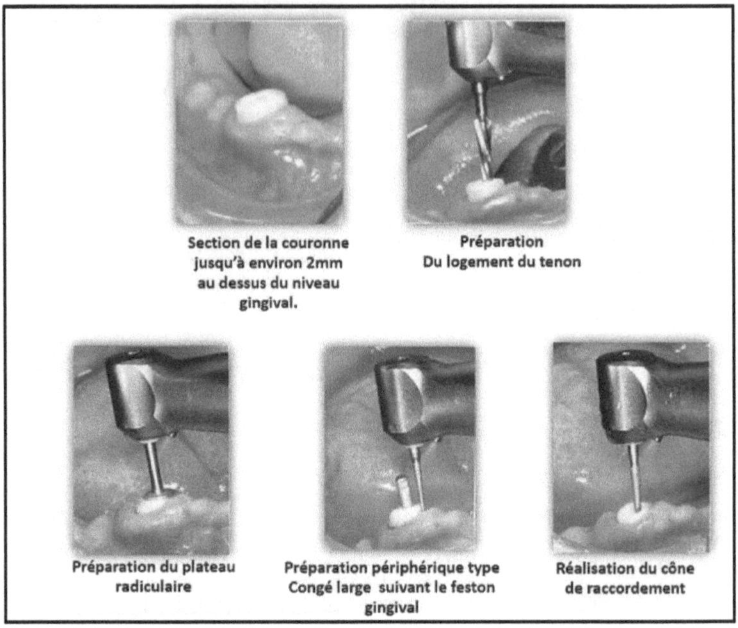

Figure 48: Richmond preparation of both canines [11]

Impression taking:

In the maxilla: Overall impression after rectification of the preparations using the wash technique (Figure 49).

Mandible: The impression had a dual purpose, as it had to take into account:

- The preparations of the roots with their posts for the fabrication of the copings with attachments.
- The osteo-mucosal support surfaces and the play of the peripheral elements.

The impression tray was a custom-made impression tray (PEI) fabricated on the plaster model after removal. The peripheral seal was achieved using polyether with traction of the cheeks and lips, opening and closing movements of the mouth, and protraction and retraction of the tongue. The impression was taken with calcinable pins in place ( ) (Figure 50).

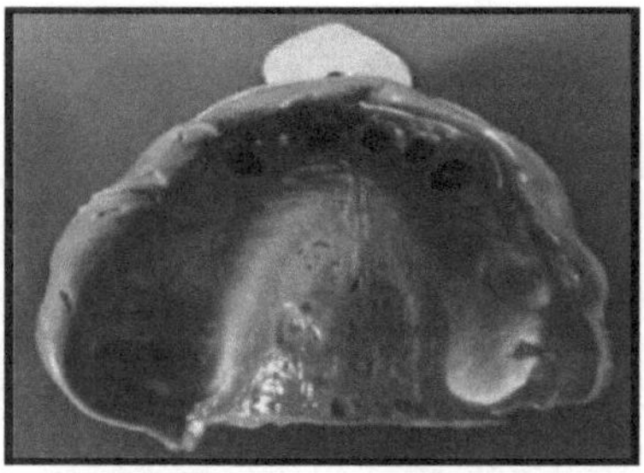

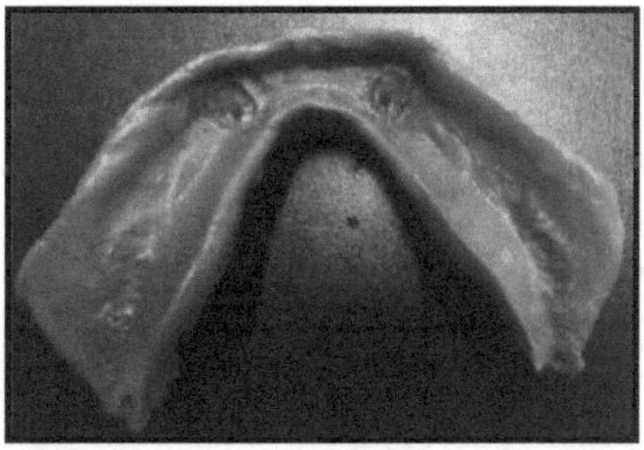

Figure 49: Full maxillary impression	Figure 50: Impression taken with pins in place in the mandible (*)

- Recording of the occlusion and placement in the articulator: this recording was used to sculpt the maxillary bridge and mandibular copings (Figure 51).

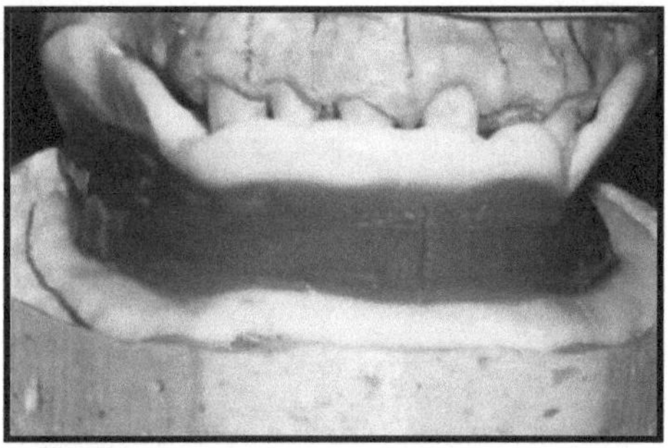

Figure 51: Recording of the mandibular-cranial relationships is performed in RC - correct DVO

- In the laboratory, two parabolic caps with pins were sculpted and secured to the anchor bar, the positioning of which was guided by silicone keys.
- The laboratory technician then cast the bar-retained overdenture system and the maxillary bridge with extra-coronal attachments.

Then, we moved on to the in-mouth try-in (Figures 52 and 53).

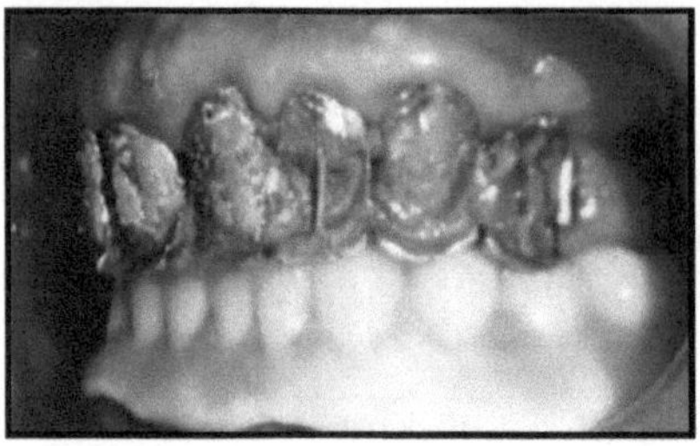

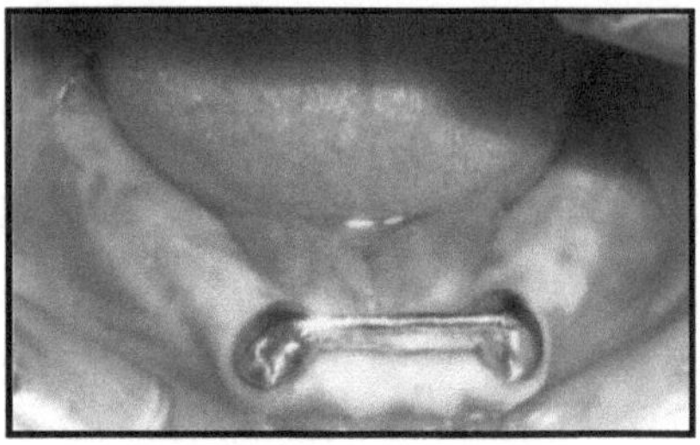

Figure 52: Try-in of the metal framework for the maxillary bridge	Figure 53: Try-in of the anchor bar in the mouth

After trying out the maxillary bridge and fitting the aesthetic veneers, we took an impression with the prosthesis in place, which was used to sculpt the maxillary frame. The support was PEI and the material was polyether, which is characterized by its rigidity after setting.

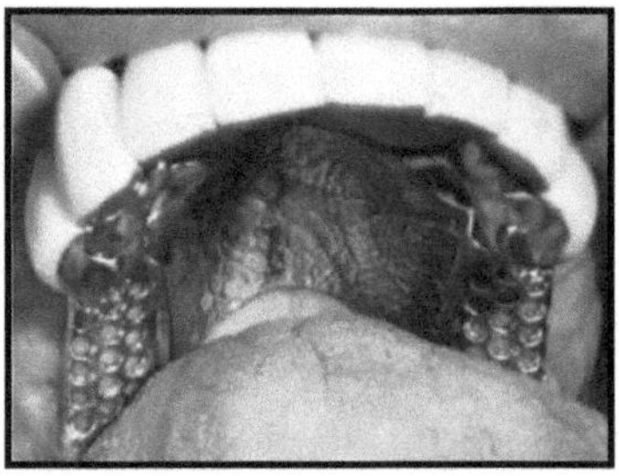

Figure 54: Trying out the frame in the mouth

- Steps in the fabrication of the complete mandibular prosthesis in the laboratory:
- The transfer riders were placed on the bar (Figure 55).
- Plaster was applied for direct polymerization on the initial model (Figure 56).
- The positioning of the flexible yellow-gold stainless steel trays ensured the perfect placement of the plastic riders (Figure 57).
- The silicone keys, taken from the pre-assembly, were put in place and used for the final assembly of the teeth.
- The model with the teeth mounted on wax was placed in a muffle for resin

polymerization. A space was left in the intrados for the placement of the riders.

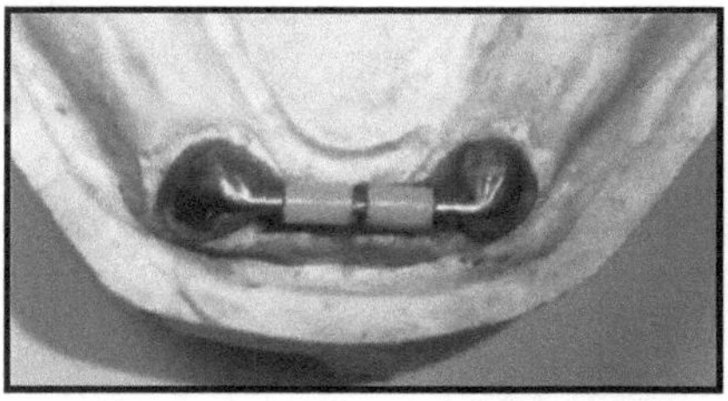

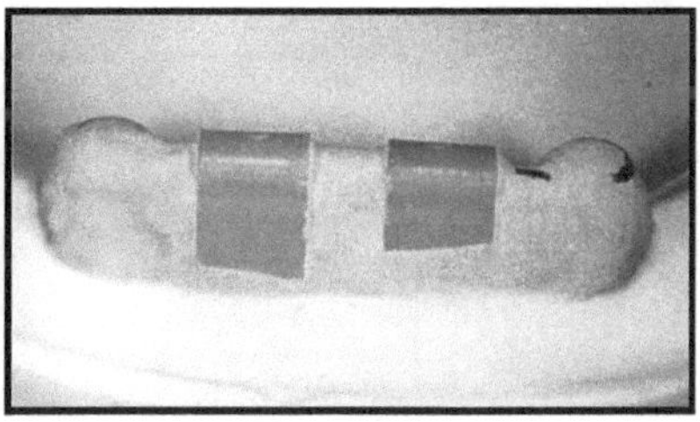

Figure 55: Placement of the transfer riders on the bar	Figure 56: Plaster discharge

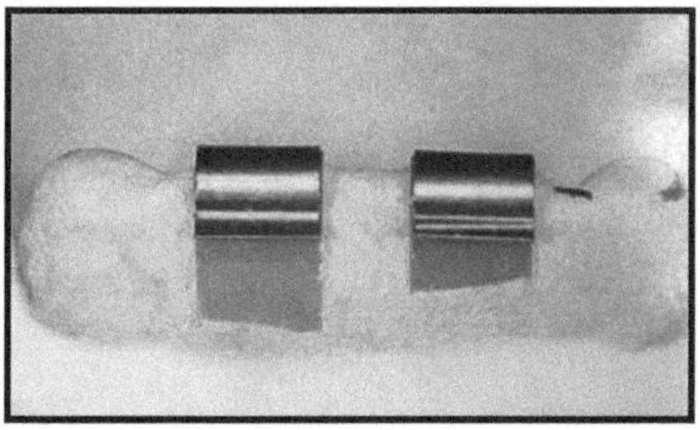

Figure 57: Positioning of flexible stainless steel stalls

- Next, we recorded the occlusion for mounting the maxillary teeth, using the maxillary frame and complete mandibular prosthesis as a support.
- Once the wax assembly had been approved, polymerization was carried out.
- On the day of insertion, the dentures were balanced in the mouth, then the bar was sealed in place and the retention clips were placed in their positions on the prosthetic intrados (Figure 58).

; regular checks in the following months would be advisable.

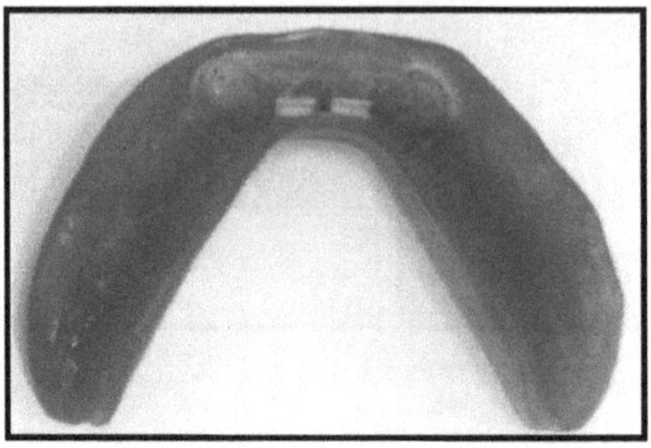

Figure 58: Sealing of retention riders in the intrados of the prosthesis

The complete supra-implant denture

The complete overdenture prosthesis (PACSI) is a simple and reliable prosthetic solution for improving prosthetic balance.
The PACSI must meet the criteria for a conventional complete denture and must guarantee stabilization and support (2, 58).
The 2002 McGill Consensus on removable implant-supported prostheses stated that (32): "Currently available evidence suggests that rehabilitation of the edentulous mandible with a conventional prosthesis is no longer the prosthetic treatment of first choice. A prosthesis retained by two symphyseal implants supporting axial attachments or connected by a connecting bar should become the first treatment option for the mandible."
PACSI is a reliable alternative to implant-supported dentures when the latter are not indicated. It is also indicated in cases of instability and/or lack of retention of conventional complete dentures.
Similarly, it is the solution of choice in patients with significant ridge resorption, hyposalivation, xerostomia, psychomotor deficits, Parkinson's disease, and uncontrolled perioral and lingual movements (82, 77).

1. Choosing the number and positions of implants

1.1. Choice of number of implants

Oral rehabilitation with implant-supported PAC is an attractive solution. However, opinions differ on the appropriate number of implants to support a mandibular PAC.
The choice of the number of implants that is appropriate for a particular clinical situation is subjective and depends on the knowledge and experience of the clinician, as well as many other factors (84).
According to the McGill consensus (32), a complete denture supported by two implants should be considered the first treatment option for an edentulous mandible.
Two implants measuring 4 mm in diameter and 8 mm in length are sufficient to achieve

the desired retention and stability. However, this decision is not suitable for all patients, and other factors must be taken into account when planning treatment (84). It is recommended to increase the number of implants in cases of significant bone resorption, increased occlusal forces, high retention requirements, or when the implants used have a length of< 8mm or a diameter of< 3.5mm. (2, 8).

1.2.Choice of implant positions in PACSI [87,84,2,56]

Ideally, implants should be located at the symphysis, on either side and equidistant from the midline, at the level of the lateral incisors/canines (87). This area has many advantages (84):

- Bone resorption is less significant than in the posterior region, with better bone quality.
- Surgery in this region is the least critical, with a success rate of over 95%.

If the implants are positioned more posteriorly (at the level of the first premolars), they form an anteroposterior axis of rotation. This axis will cause significant tilting of the prosthesis around the implants, and the attachments will concentrate the stresses even more (87).

The anterior mandibular region can be divided into five equal zones, in which 2 or 4 implants could be positioned. This allows implants to be added if the removable prosthesis supported by two implants needs to be replaced by a prosthesis supported by four implants. Similarly, if a fifth median implant is indicated in the presence of a PACSI with four implants (84).

The implants must be positioned symmetrically and parallel to each other to prevent premature wear of the attachment components and to protect the implants from excessive stress (2).

The attachment system chosen also dictates the position of the implants (56):

- In the case of axial attachments, the implants can be placed close together: the practitioner must take into account the diameter of the female part and the thickness of the resin required to hold the female part in the PACSI, i.e. 5 to 6 mm.

If three implants are placed, they must be straight (Figure 64b). Three axial attachments, placed on three non-straight implants, prevent angular play of the prosthesis. The central implant then receives excessive stress (Figure 64c).

If four implants are placed, they must be symmetrical in relation to the median sagittal plane with strict parallelism between the four implants. (Figure 64d)

- In the case of a bar: the implants are connected by a bar, which should ideally be parallel to the frontal plane (Figure 64e).

If four implants are placed, they form a trapezoid and must be symmetrical in relation to the median sagittal plane (Figure 64f).

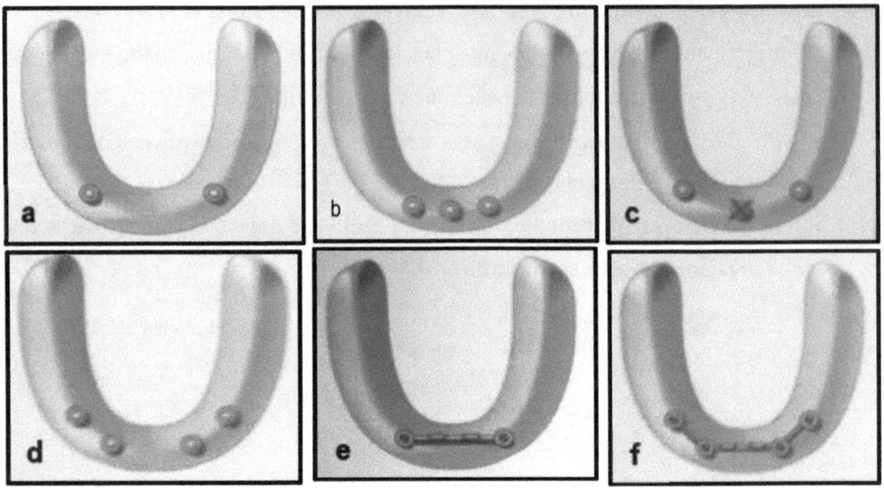

Figure 64: Implant positions in the mandible in PACSI

(a) Two implants symmetrical in relation to the median sagittal plane, covered with two axial attachments (b) Three aligned implants, covered with axial attachments (c) Three non-aligned implants: unfavorable biomechanical situation (d) Four implants symmetrical in relation to the median sagittal plane

(e) A straight bar connecting two implants (f) Four symmetrical implants connected by three bar segments

2. PACSI attachment systems

Spherical attachments and connecting bars are widely used in PACSI, resilient attachments and telescopic caps can also be used, whereas magnetic attachments are no longer recommended (83, 58).

It is important to note that in PACSI, support and stabilization are provided by the prosthesis; implants and attachments contribute to secondary retention.

In order to comply with this rule, the attachment system must allow axial play to enable vertical translation, as well as angular play to allow distal rotation. This ensures that mucosal depressibility is maintained (56).

Axial attachments and anchor bars offer this relative freedom of movement, whereas the telescopic system, due to its rigidity, does not allow any movement.

In the case of implant-supported PACs, which are completely different from mucosal PACs, a specific attachment system is used. It is characterized by its lack of freedom of movement, its rigidity, and its shape, which prevents any rotation. It can be either a rectangular bar with riders or a bar/counter bar with axial attachments or riders incorporated into the bar.

For this type of prosthesis, retention, stabilization, and support are entirely provided by the implant system (71, 64).

2.1. Criteria for choosing attachment systems

No single attachment system can be chosen for all clinical situations. The practitioner must consider various general and specific parameters in order to select the appropriate attachment system.

Table III: Technical and clinical requirements for attachment systems (13)

Requirements	– Small dimensions/minimal space requirements (in terms of **vertical and horizontal directions)** vertical and horizontal) Wear resistance Easy replacement of worn parts Possibility of corrections in case of discrepancies between natural and implant pillar axes
Clinical requirements planning and implementation	:– Adjustable retention – Easy handling when fixing the female parts by – self-curing resin – Versatile range of applications (ubiquitous) – Cost-effectiveness
Clinical requirements: follow-up and subsequent care	– Adequate oral hygiene possible – Retention elements can be easily activated – Reduced investment for maintenance procedures – Simple handling

Unlike in the maxilla, implant fixation is not mandatory in the mandible; other parameters must be taken into account.

❖ Forms **the alveolar ridge (58,84,1)**

A straight anterior ridge (U-shaped arch) or a very slightly curved ridge points to a connecting bar, and axial attachments may also be indicated.

In the case of a rounded ridge (V-shaped arch), the use of a curved bar with two implants may create an unfavorable lever arm. By reducing the curvature, it may encroach on the tongue space and impair function. In this case, either axial attachments should be chosen or additional implants should be added so that the curvature is divided into several straight segments compatible with the use of the bar (Figure 66).

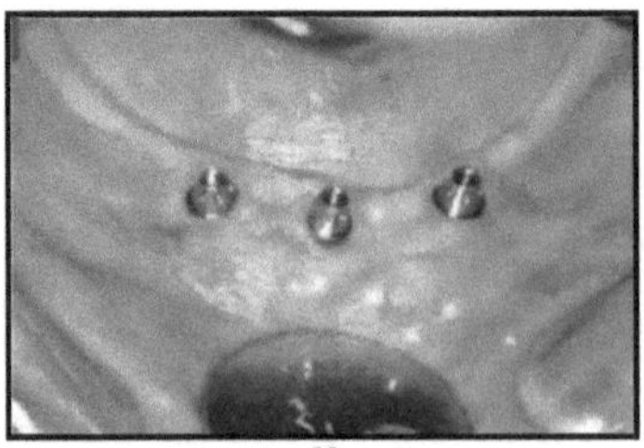

Figure 66: Placement of three mandibular implants for a connecting bar (86)

❖ **The inter-implant distance (84,58)**

A good distance between adjacent implants must be considered. In the case of a bar, 8 to 10 mm between the proximal faces of the implants is necessary for the placement of at least one abutment on the bar without deformation.

❖ **Resorption level and bone quality (86)**

Weak bone structures encourage us to increase the number of supporting implants or even to connect them using a connecting bar.

Some authors recommend the use of four implants joined together in cases where bone height is less than 12 mm.

❖ **Available prosthetic space (29,84,8)**

The prosthetic space is estimated using positioning keys or guides in the horizontal and vertical directions (29).

When vertical space is limited, the use of a bar may violate the interocclusal space. The bar requires a minimum of 12 mm between the crest and the incisal edge. For spherical attachments, the minimum vertical space required is 10-12 mm and for the Locator, 8.5 mm.

In the horizontal direction, the buccolingual space must be taken into account, and the attachment must be placed on the crest of the ridge to achieve its best biomechanical benefits (84).

Failure to comply with the prosthetic space may result in an overcontoured prosthesis, excessive VDO, loss of attachment, and even prosthesis fracture (8).

❖ **Implant parallelism (86,56,1,83)**

Implants must be as parallel as possible. Lack of parallelism between two PACSI-bearing implants may lead to premature wear of the attachment systems or even loss of osseointegration in the event of parasitic forces (86).

Axial attachments have a degree of axis correction limited to around ten degrees in general (up to 20 degrees for the Locator system); bars are more tolerant (56).

This lack of parallelism can, in some situations, be compensated for by angled attachments or Locator®. The male part of the Locator® has an automatic alignment function. It can correct implant axis divergence of up to 40° without any significant negative effect on retention

(inserts with central pin) (1, 83).

❖ **Other factors** [29,84]

- Immediate loading of the implant indicates the use of a connecting bar. The bar ensures the primary stability necessary for osseointegration of the implants.
- The cost of treatment and the cost of repairs must be taken into account when developing the treatment plan, and the patient must be informed of these costs.
- The connecting bar and telescopic attachments are more expensive than other attachments.
- The amount of retention required: the connecting bar provides more retention than axial attachments.
- Factors such as patient expectations, the knowledge and skills of the dentist and laboratory technicians, and the opposing maxillary arch may play a role in the selection of the attachment and type of prosthesis.

Table IV: Criteria for choosing between bars and axial attachments [80]

Criteria	Axial attachments	Connection bars
Implant parallelism	Strict (tolerance 5 to 15°)	Axis adjustment possible
Prosthetic volume	Low	Significant
Inter-implant distance	Not important	Minimum 15 mm for two cavalier
Shape of the arch	Any	Straight anterior arch
Implant position	IL/C/PM Symmetrical in relation to the midline	Rather incisivo-canine

2.2.Influence of the opposing arch [56]

When facing a maxillary arch with natural teeth or teeth restored with fixed prostheses, a mandibular PACSI will be subjected to greater stress than if two PACSIs are opposed to each other or if the maxillary arch is restored with a PAC. When both arches have removable prostheses, the occlusal stresses will be transferred to the depressible mucosa of both arches. On the other hand, a PACSI opposed to a fixed prosthesis or natural teeth will receive almost all of the forces, since the movements tolerated by the mucosa are greater than those tolerated by the desmodont.

In this case, the choice of attachment will be oriented towards a system that is more or less tolerant in terms of the freedom of movement of the PACSI.

2.3. The use of mini-implants (41,40,84,61)

This solution is an interesting alternative for mandibular prosthesis stability when conventional implants cannot be used. Mini-implants are characterized by a diameter of less than 3 mm.

This technique involves placing four mini-implants in the mandible (Figure 68). The surgery to insert the mini-implants is simple and quick. The mini-implants are self-tapping and require only a single drill. In addition, this technique does not require a flap, making it less invasive and very reassuring for elderly patients. Mini implants can be loaded immediately or after a period of time. Immediate loading allows for the restoration of comfort, aesthetics, and chewing function. Its success rate is over 95%, comparable to that of delayed loading.

The success rate of this technique is closely linked to the spatial distribution of the implants and the method of connection between the prosthesis and the implant (41, 40).

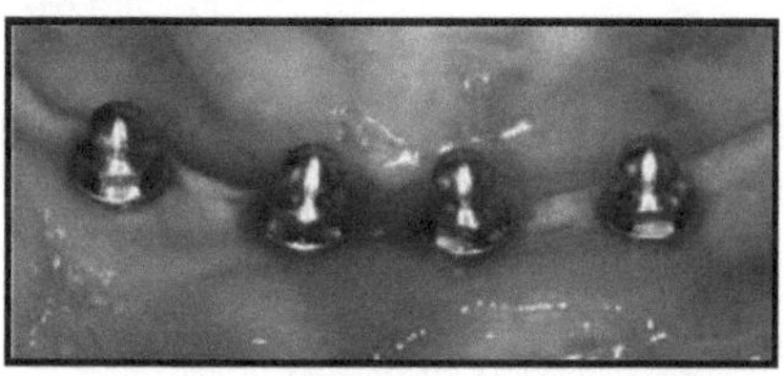

Figure 68: Intraoral view of mini-implants with their axial attachments (40)

2.3.1. Advantages (84,40)

- Mini implants can be placed in narrow sites with limited bone height.
- The surgery to place mini-implants is minimally invasive. The healing period is shorter than for conventional implants, with reduced post-operative complications.

- Immediate loading.
- Treatment at a reasonable cost.
- Improvement of various oral functions.

2.3.2. Disadvantages (40,61)

- The placement of mini-implants is not an easy procedure; on the contrary, it requires an experienced practitioner. The use of a single drill bit means that the implant axis must be correct from the outset for all mini-implants to avoid any parallelism issues.
- The male part of the attachment cannot be replaced if worn, when they are made of a single piece.
- In addition to the complications of standard implant systems, there is a greater risk of fracture with mini-implants due to their small diameter and design.

3. Comparison between PACSI and PACSR ( )

3.1. Similarities between PACSR and PACSI (82,77,17,74)

3.1.1. advantages

- Both techniques offer better prosthetic balance thanks to improved retention and stability compared to conventional dentures.
- Improved quality of life for patients through improved chewing, speech, and swallowing.
- Chewing efficiency is higher for overdentures than for conventional dentures. The difference between PACSI and PACSR is insignificant.
- Maintaining bone capital limits resorption.
- Less BMD loss than with conventional prostheses.

3.1.2. : disadvantages

- PACSI and PACSR are two removable solutions that are more expensive than conventional prostheses.
- The treatment period and number of sessions required are longer than with conventional techniques.
- The presence of attachment systems requires rigorous hygiene.

- There is a high rate of prosthesis fracture.
- Regular check-ups are required for prosthesis maintenance and reactivation of attachment systems.

3.1.3. Indications

- The abutments must not be unilateral.
- Sufficient prosthetic space is required for the attachment system to be placed.
- Use of articulated attachments that can accommodate the difference in tissue depressibility between the fibromucosa and the abutment.
- It is essential to have a conventional prosthesis that complies with best practice.

3.2. The difference between the two techniques (82,77,27,74,17)

- Prosthesis cushioning:

The vertical sinking of the prosthesis is less significant when using implants than with natural roots.

The application of a lateral force on the tooth causes it to rotate around the hypomochlion. However, at the implant level, this force causes cratering around the implant neck and then fracture of the implant.

- The presence of the alveolar ligament, in the context of PACSR, ensures the proper transfer of occlusal forces to the alveolar bone. Proprioception prevents occlusal overload and bone resorption due to excessive forces. The implant is ankylosed: osseo .

- Discrimination ability, which is the ability to distinguish between different stimuli depending on periodontal receptors, is higher when the overdenture is supported by a tooth root than by an implant.
- A significant decrease in electromyographic activity of the masseter muscles and an increase in temporal muscle activity in patients rehabilitated with PACSR, compared to conventional complete dentures and PACSI.
- The lifespan of PACSR is patient-dependent. For PACSI, it depends on the implant surgery, the loading protocol, and the pre-prosthetic and prosthetic stages.

4. Illustration

A 65-year-old female patient with old removable prostheses consulted the removable partial denture department at the Monastir dental clinic. She complained of mandibular prosthetic instability during chewing and phonation.

4.1. Clinical examination and radiographic

Clinical examination:

On extraoral examination, facial symmetry, equal facial planes, a straight mouth opening, and moderately developed musculature were noted.

The intraoral examination revealed subtotal maxillary edentulism, with residual teeth 22 and 23, and total mandibular edentulism (Figure 69).

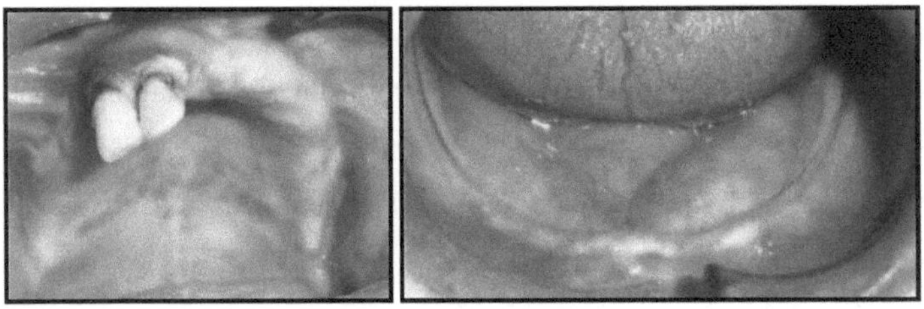

Figure 69: Initial condition of both arches

Examination of the osteomucosal surfaces showed that the mandible had a knife-edge ridge covered by a thin fibromucosa.

In the maxilla, the crest was moderately high, and the tuberosities were erased.

Radiological examination:

The panoramic radiograph showed an unfavorable CR/RR ratio at the level of the persistent teeth (Figure 70).

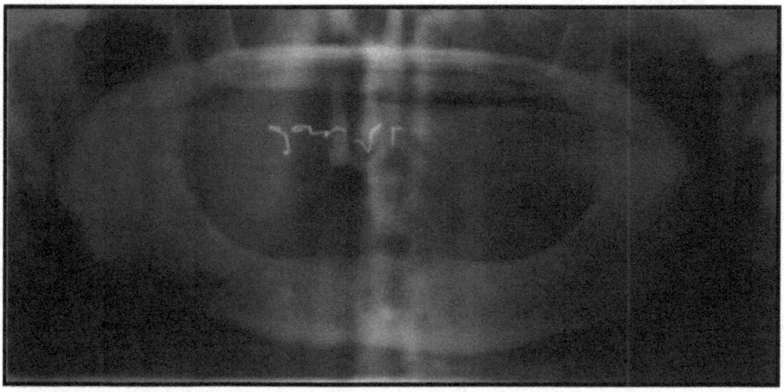

Figure 70: Panoramic radiograph (*)

Occlusion examination:

The DVO was lost, the PIM was not preserved, and the study casts on articulators showed sufficient HOPU.

4.2. -preprosthetic treatment

Extraction of residual maxillary teeth.

4.3. Prosthetic diagnosis

This is a case of complete edentulism in the maxilla (Sangiuolo class II) and complete edentulism in the mandible (Sangiuolo class III).

- Occlusal diagnosis:
- Occlusal plan to be established
- PIM absent
- DVO collapsed
- HOPU sufficient
- Anterior guide absent

4.4. Prosthetic decision

- Complete maxillary denture.
- Prosthesis denture complete mandibular stabilized by two

symphyseal implant to improve retention.

4.5. Prosthetic steps

Fabrication of complete maxillary and mandibular prostheses:

Table V: Prosthetic fabrication sequence

At the clinic	*In the laboratory*
1- Taking primary impressions.	➔ Casting of impressions and preparation of PEIs.
2- Taking secondary impressions.	➔ Casting of an d production of bases occlusion
3- Recording of the occlusion in RC-DVO placement in articulator and selection of prosthetic teeth.	➔ Mounting of teeth on correct wax,
4- Trying out the wax setup	➔ Placing in the mold
5- Insertion into the mouth and occlusal adjustment of the prostheses.	

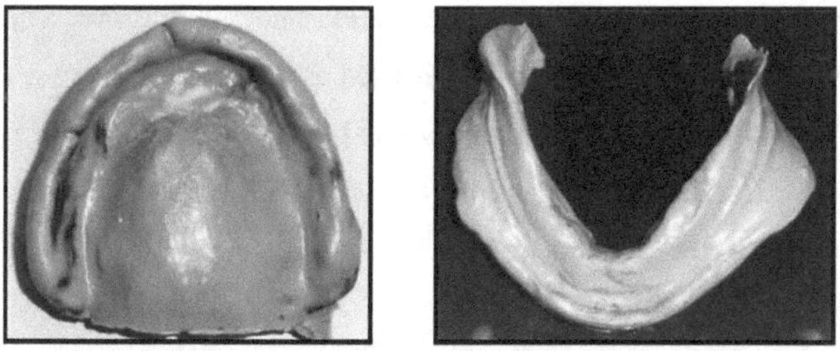

Figure 71: Secondary maxillary and mandibular impressions (*)

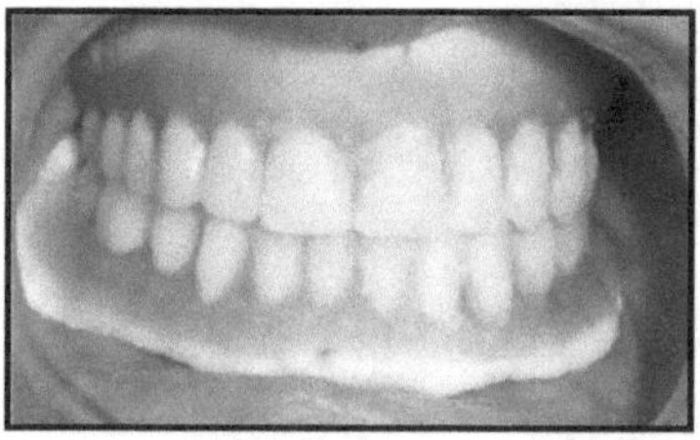

Figure 72: Trying out the waxassembly

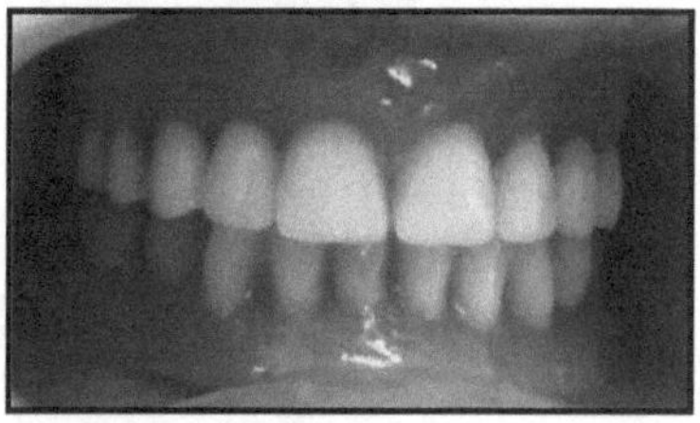

Figure 73: Trying out the prostheses

Cone Beam scan:

To assess the feasibility of implant treatment and select the implants, a cone beam was performed. The mandibular prosthesis was used as a radiological guide (Figure 74). The data collected from the Cone Beam guided us towards choosing implants with a diameter of Ø= 3.75 mm and a length of L=10 mm, given the narrow width of the ridge and the proximity of the mental nerve.

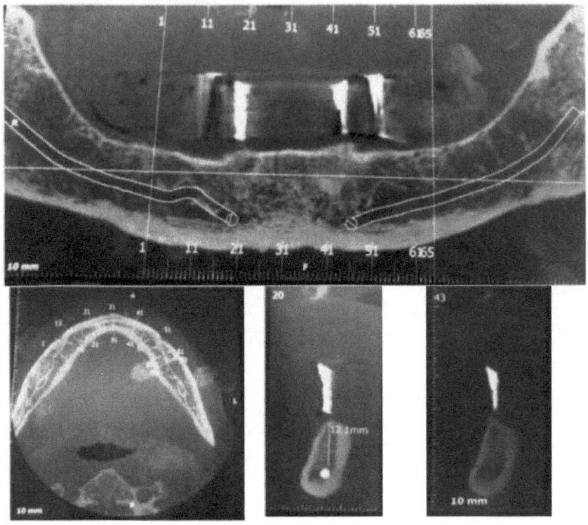

Figure 74: Cone beam radiograph allowing selection of implant diameter and length (*)

Surgical phase:

- Incision at the crest and detachment of the vestibular and lingual flaps (Figure 75).
- Positioning of the surgical guide and drilling of the first site in the correct sequence. The depth of the drilling was checked using a graduated gauge.
- Positioning of the direction indicator, then drilling of the second site, ensuring parallelism between the two (Figure 77).
- Insertion of implants and cover screws, then repositioning of the flap and suturing (Figures 78 and 79).
- Prescription of an antibiotic, a corticosteroid, and a painkiller

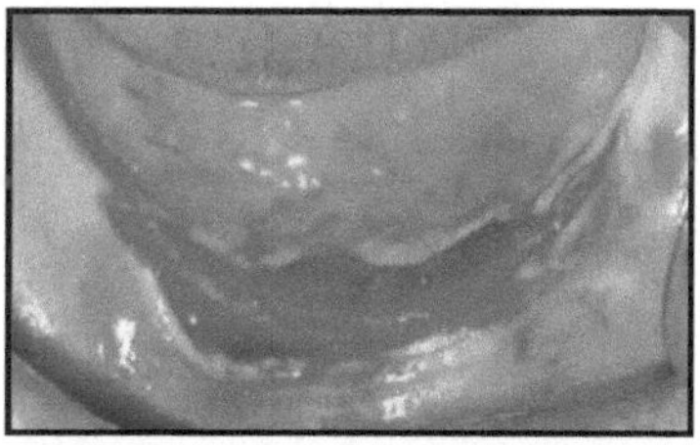

Figure 75: Incision at the top of the crest and detachment of the flaps (*)

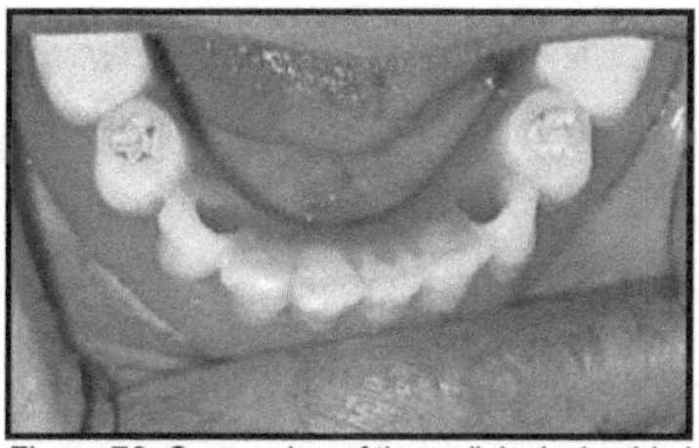

Figure 76: Conversion of the radiological guide into a surgical guide

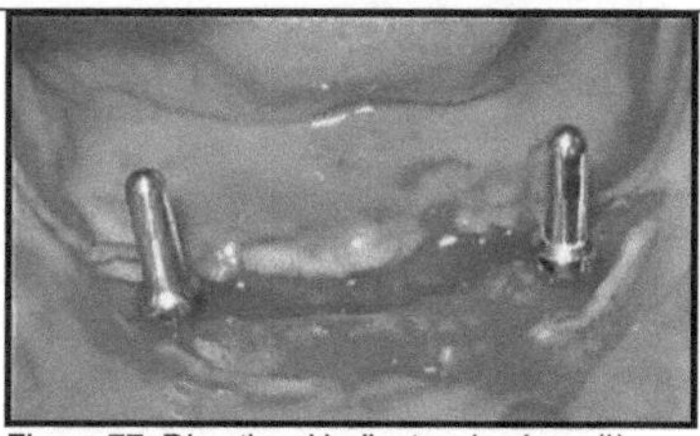

Figure 77: Directional indicators in place (*)

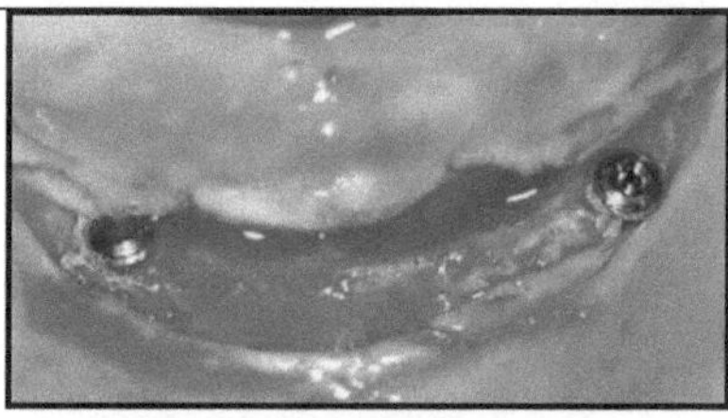

Figure 78: Protection of implants with cover screws (*)

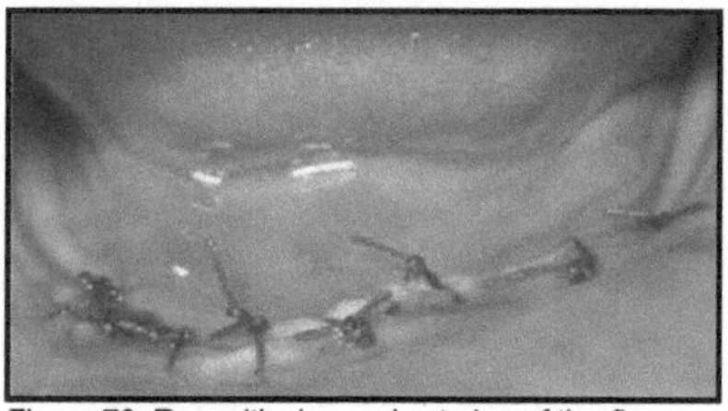

Figure 79: Repositioning and suturing of the flap

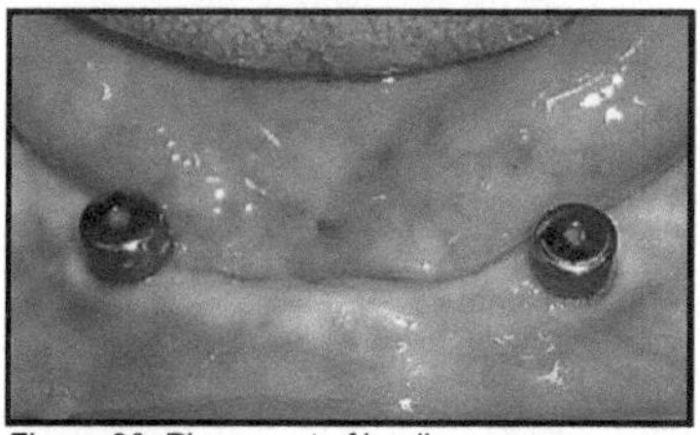

Figure 80: Placement of healing screws

- After 3 months of bone healing (osseointegration phase), the cover screws were removed and the healing screws were placed (Figure 80). Mucosal healing would take 6 to 8 weeks.
- A control X-ray was taken to check the quality of the fit between the abutment and the implant.

Prosthetic phase:

After mucosal healing, the practitioner removed the healing screws. He then attached the male parts of the ball attachments to the implants (Figure 81). Once the male part was in place, the female part was attached on top (Figure 82). Spacer rings separated the two parts to ensure a certain amount of resilience.

The mandibular prosthesis was hollowed out at the implant sites, then filled with self-curing resin and placed in the mouth (Figure 83). The resin was set under occlusal pressure (Figure 84). Finishing was carried out after complete polymerization (Figure 85). After polishing, the practitioner taught the patient how to insert and remove her prosthesis and explained the necessary instructions for maintaining the prostheses. Regular check-ups would be necessary to assess the osseointegration of the implants and the integrity of the attachment system.

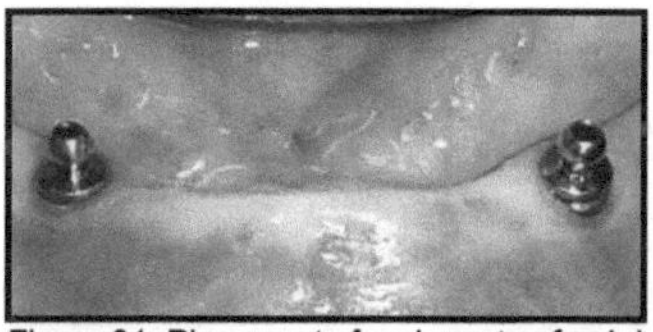

Figure 81: Placement of male parts of axial attachments

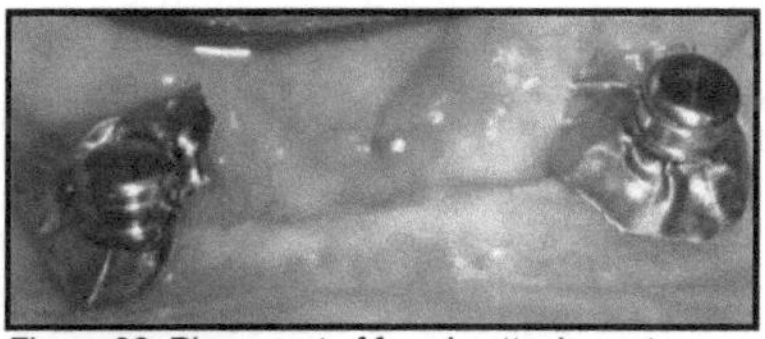

Figure 82: Placement of female attachments

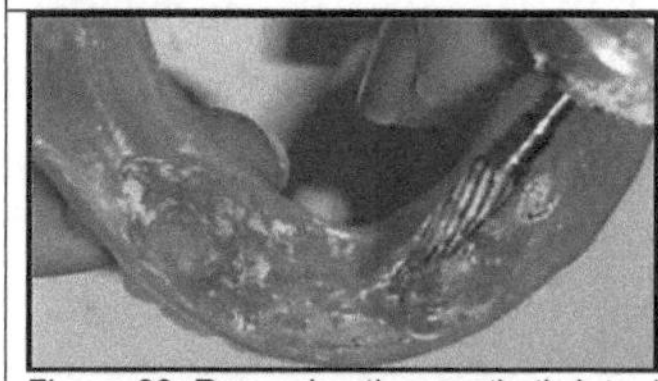

Figure 83: Recessing the prosthetic intaglio surface and filling with self-curing resin

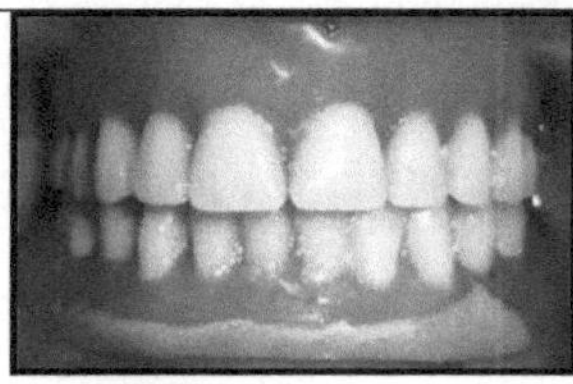

Figure 84: The patient remains in occlusion while the resin sets

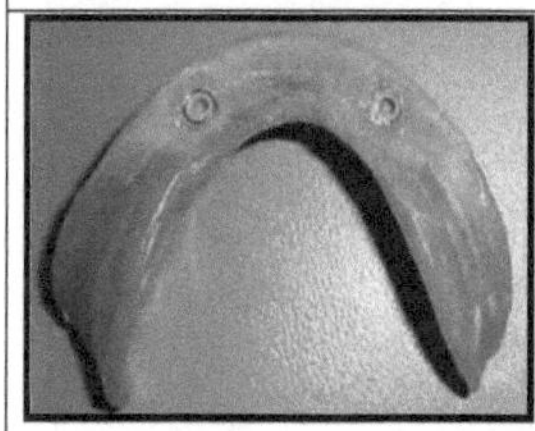

Figure 85: Female parts of the attachment in the prosthetic intrados

During follow-up visits, the patient reported a marked improvement in chewing efficiency and complete satisfaction with the aesthetic appearance of the dentures.

The use of implants has limited resorption in this patient, optimized retention, stability, and various oral functions, and has undoubtedly improved comfort and quality of life thanks to better psychological integration (2, 82).

A systematic review conducted by Kutkut. A et al (49) comparing conventional complete dentures with dentures retained by non-integrated implants showed a clear improvement in patient satisfaction and masticatory function with implant-supported dentures.

Table VI: Summary table of ways to optimize complete mandibular dentures

Means of optimization	Principle	Objectives
Pre-prosthetic surgery	Maximizing the use of anatomical areas improves the support and retention of the prosthesis. Surgery results in a better anatomical environment.	- Correction of anatomical or pathological conditions that prevent optimal prosthetic function. - Enlargement of the prosthetic support area.
Tissue conditioning	This is a treatment designed to prepare the oral tissues for receiving a prosthesis. It uses a MECT material, delivered via a removable prosthesis (old or newly designed).	- Restore the viscoelasticity of the fibromucosa and achieve a clinically healthy appearance. - Extension of the prosthetic support surface. - Optimization of the biofunctional space volume.
Piezography	Piezography is the molding of a plastic mass by intrinsic pressures generated by the peri-prosthetic muscle masses	- Optimization of stability. - Achieving better prosthetic integration. - Greater freedom during functions. - Improved aesthetics. - Easy prosthetic hygiene.
Stabilizing polished surfaces	Stabilizing polished surfaces are areas on the prosthetic extrados that allow the paraprosthetic musculature to participate in the balance of the prosthesis. Stabilizing polished surfaces are obtained either by sculpting the wax or using specific piezographic impression techniques.	- Better prosthesis retention. - Use of paraprosthetic musculature to improve prosthetic balance. - Improved aesthetics.
Adhesives	This is a therapeutic supplement applied to the inner surface of a removable prosthesis to temporarily improve retention and stability.	Achieve patient comfort and satisfaction through improved retention and stability, reduced prosthesis movement during use.
PACSR	Preserving residual tooth roots with good endodontic and periodontal value improves the retention and stability of mandibular PACs. Thanks to their strategic positions, the two mandibular canines are the most commonly used teeth.	- Preservation of periodontal proprioception and neuromuscular coordination. - Maintenance of alveolar bone capital. - Improved prognosis for PAC through better stability and retention.
PACSI	According to the McGill consensus, a prosthesis retained by two symphyseal implants is the first choice of treatment for the mandible.	- Improved masticatory efficiency - Prevention of bone loss - Optimization of retention, stability, and various oral functions. - Improved patient comfort and quality of life.

Role of post-prosthetic maintenance

After fitting, it is important to ensure the maximum longevity of the denture. The dentist must provide the patient with several tips to guarantee the best use of their denture. They must explain hygiene advice and recommend an effective method for cleaning dentures.

It is important to advise the patient to remove the dentures at night. This protects the supporting tissues, ensures better blood circulation, and maintains the health of the oral tissues.

Similarly, practitioners must emphasize the need for periodic follow-up visits after the prosthesis has been fitted to check its fit, the effectiveness of the patient's cleaning routine, and the condition of the soft tissues. Patients with complete removable dentures believe that because they have no natural teeth, regular visits to the dentist are unnecessary and therefore only visit the dentist when they need a new denture, or if the dentures are broken or worn.

Patients should also be aware that the prosthesis has a limited lifespan and may need to be replaced after 4 to 5 years (24).

There are two approaches to maintaining removable dental prostheses: a personal approach and a professional approach.

- The patient: their role is to maintain adequate oral hygiene and clean the removable prosthesis, follow the instructions for use provided by the practitioner, and attend maintenance appointments as scheduled (24).
- The practitioner checks hygiene, occlusion balance, and prosthetic base rehabilitation. If necessary, the prosthetic base must be relined to compensate for any changes in the alveolar ridge. (2)

1. Cleaning of dentures (33)

Felton et al (33) have compiled guidelines for cleaning dentures:

1. Daily thorough removal of biofilm from the oral cavity and complete dentures is of paramount importance in minimizing denture stomatitis and contributing to good oral and general health.

2. To reduce levels of biofilm, potentially harmful bacteria, and fungi, patients should do the following:

- Dentures should be cleaned daily by soaking and brushing with an effective, non-abrasive cleaner.
- Denture cleaners should only be used outside the mouth.
- Dentures should be thoroughly rinsed after soaking and brushing before being reinserted into the mouth.

3. Dentures should undergo periodic professional cleaning using ultrasonic cleaners to minimize biofilm buildup over time. Professional cleaning may use ultrasound or microwave irradiation.
4. Dentures should never be placed in boiling water.
5. Prostheses should not be soaked in sodium hypochlorite bleach or products containing sodium hypochlorite for periods longer than 10 minutes.

2. Repair of prosthetic bases (81)

Repairing the prosthetic base involves creating a new resin base in the prosthetic intrados while preserving the occlusion and tooth alignment. This may be indicated for new or old dentures. However, these dentures must not have any aesthetic defects or intermaxillary or occlusal problems.

There are two types:

- A total restoration of the denture base using a thermopolymerizable acrylic resin.
- Partial restoration allowing superficial rehabilitation of the denture, carried out with a self-polymerizing resin. This can be done either directly in the mouth, but the setting reaction is exothermic, or indirectly by passing through a laboratory stage.

In the event of total or partial restoration carried out in the laboratory, the practitioner takes an impression using the existing prosthesis. This is an occlusal pressure impression, known as a "tertiary" or "supplementary" impression.

2.1. Indications [81]

- Lack of stability of the prosthesis leading to loss of retention.
- In the presence of errors in the registration of the support surface, during the fabrication of the prosthesis or due to modifications made by the practitioner in order to resolve the patient's complaints.
- Pathological or physiological alteration of the support surfaces.
- Improving aesthetics: In fact, restoration only affects the false gum. Restoring the base ensures support for the paraprosthetic tissues and corrects any damage caused by wear, fracture, or lack of resin thickness.
- Alteration of the surface condition of the resin, promoting bacterial colonization.

2.2. Contraindications [81]

- Lack of occlusal balance
- Incorrect recording of intermaxillary relationships
- Erroneous positioning or orientation of the occlusal plane
- Significantly overestimated vertical dimension of occlusion
- Failure to comply with tooth mounting rules and invasion of the prosthetic corridor.

3. Special featuresof the complete implant-supported denture (56,85,29,2)

Maintenance appointments take place one week after the PACSI is fitted, then after one month, six months, and once a year. They are more frequent during the first year of use (56, 85).

During the maintenance session, the dentist must check the implant-tooth-prosthesis balance on three levels (29):

- At the bone level using X-rays: check osseointegration and cratering around the implants.
- At the gingival level: check for plaque and the condition of the peri-implant tissues.
- At the occlusal level: check the occlusion.

The practitioner also works on the peri-implant gingiva when loosening screws, treating fractures, and relining. In the event of loss of retention, the practitioner must replace or activate the retention clip or the female part of the attachment (Figure 86).
The spherical abutment can also be replaced in case of wear (2).

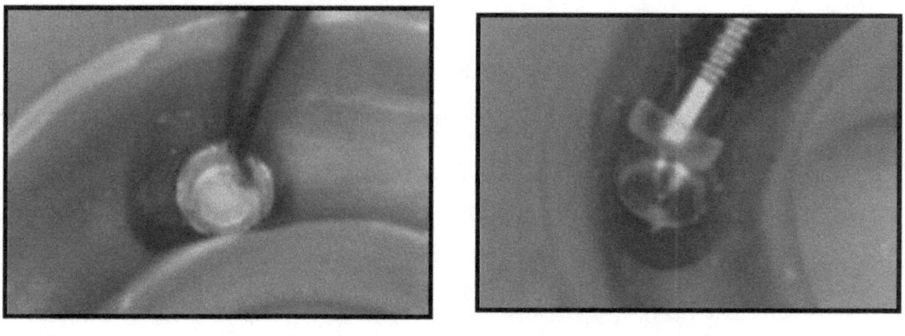

Figure 86: Replacement of the nylon attachment on the Locator system

Conclusion

Despite revolutionary advances in prevention and care, total edentulism remains a common condition. Practitioners frequently see patients with complete edentulism in the mandibular arches. Achieving prosthetic stability is
perceived at the time as a challenge to be overcome: unlike the maxilla, where the presence of the palate provides a good support surface, the mandibular support surface is reduced by the presence of the tongue. In addition, advanced resorption of the edentulous ridges combined with the relative migration of the mylohyoid and buccinator muscle insertions toward the top of the residual ridge, as well as the highly destabilizing horizontal forces developed by the paraprosthetic musculature, make this context unfavorable for achieving mandibular PAC equilibrium. Mandibular PAC is generally unstable and non-retentive.
Several techniques and methods are available to dentists to improve and overcome the difficulties encountered.
Pre-prosthetic surgery and tissue conditioning are two interesting techniques that can improve the anatomical environment and achieve healthy tissue.
During the fabrication of a complete mandibular prosthesis, every step must contribute to improving the retention and stability of the prosthesis.
Piezography can be a valuable aid. It allows complete dentures to be fabricated in harmony with the specific anatomy and physiology of each edentulous patient.
The use of a balanced occlusion, whether conventional or lingualized, significantly increases the stability of the prosthesis during use.
Adhesives for removable prostheses, despite being rarely prescribed by dentists, are also considered a useful therapeutic adjunct when used appropriately. They ensure better stability and retention of the prosthesis.
The combination of the above measures is very advantageous.
It should also be noted that the use of remaining tooth roots is an interesting therapeutic option. A complete supra-radicular removable prosthesis improves stabilization,

support, and retention when combined with attachment systems. It promotes bone preservation, chewing efficiency, and psychological adaptation.

When financial resources are available, the use of osseointegrated implants is a reliable solution in most clinical situations.

References

1. **Abdelkaoui A, Berrada S, Fajri L, Abdedine A, Merzouk N.**

Attachment Locator®: step-by-step clinical instructions for use in complete removable prostheses stabilized on implants.

Actual Odonto-Stomatol 2016;280:p5

2. **Abdelkaoui A, Fajri L, Abdedine A.**

Natural roots and implants for prosthetic balance in complete removable prostheses.

Cah Prothèse 2012;159:51-59.

3. **Abdelkoui A, Lakhssassi N, Merzouk N, Berrada S.**

Complete removable prosthesis retained by a median symphyseal implant.

J Stomatol Oral Maxillofac Surg 2017;118(2):132-135

4. **Abduo J.**

Occlusal schemes for complete dentures: a systematic review.

Int J Prosthodont 2013;26:26–33.

5. **Abid A.**

The contribution of root preservation in cases of subtotal mandibular edentulism [Thesis].

Monastir: Faculty of Dental Medicine of Monastir, 2011.

6. **Adisman I K.**

The use of denture adhesives as an aid to denture treatment.

The Journal of Prosthetic Dentistry 1989;62:711-6.

7. **Alsabeeha N, Payne AGT, De Silva RK, Swain MV.**

Mandibular single-implant overdentures: A review with surgical and prosthodontic perspectives of a novel approach.

Clin Oral Impl Res. 2009;20:356–365.

8. **Bansal S, Aras MA, Chitre V.**

Guidelines for treatment planning of mandibular implant overdenture.

J Dent Implant 2014;4:86-90.

9. **Benhammou J, Yasukawa K, Juras C.**

Adhesives in removable prostheses: contribution to rules for proper use and prescription.
Prosthetic Strategy 2017;17(5):359-365.

10. Bernhardt M, Joerger R, Leize M, Azuelos A, Bourguignon S, Iskandar S.
Piezography and occlusal planning in complete dentures.
Prosthetic Synergy 2001;3(2):129-37.

11. Borel JC, Schittly J, Exbrayat J.
Manual of removable partial dentures (2nd edition).
Paris: Masson, 1994.

12. Bouraoui S, Mansour L, Trabelsi M, Chater M.
Use of natural and artificial roots in removable prostheses: Clinical cases.
African Journal of Dentistry and Implantology 2015;5

13. Büttel AE, Bühler NM, Marinello CP.
Locator® or spherical anchorage? Comparative evaluation as an aid to clinical decision-making.
Rev Mens Suisse Odonto stomatol 2009;119:910-18.

14. Cagna DR, Massad JJ, Schiesser FJ.
The neutral zone revisited: From historical concepts to modern application.
J Prosthet Dent 2009;101:405-412.

15. Carlsson GE.
Implant and root supported overdentures - a literature review and some data on bone loss in edentulous jaws.
J Adv Prosthodont 2014;6(4):245-52.

16. Chanty B.
Management and optimization of complete removable dentures in the elderly: concepts and precepts [thesis].
Nancy: Faculty of Dentistry, 2016.

17. Chen L, Xie Q, Feng H, Lin Y, Li J.
The masticatory efficiency of mandibular implant-supported overdentures as compared with tooth-supported overdentures and complete dentures.
Journal of Oral Implantology 2002;28:238-43.

18. Cherni L.

Hyperplasia in removable prostheses: origin and management [thesis].

Monastir: Faculty of Dental Medicine of Monastir, 2015.

19. Chevalier L.

Contribution of piezographic techniques to daily practice in complete removable prosthetics [thesis].

Nancy: Faculty of Dentistry, 2007.

20. Clarke P, Leven J, Youngson CC.

Managing the Unstable Mandibular Complete Denture– Tooth Placement and the Polished Surface.

Dent Update 2016;43:660–670.

21. Çomut AA, Somohano T.

Surgical and prosthetic management of a complex edentulous patient for fabrication of complete dentures.

The New York State Dental Journal 2015;81(2):29-33.

22. Cooper LF. (25)

The current and future treatment of edentulism.

Journal of Prosthodontics 2009;18:116–122

23. Cordioli G, Majzoub Z, Castagna S.

Mandibular overdentures anchored to single implants: a five-year prospective study.

J Prosthet Dent 1997;78(2):159–65.

24. Deise Osmaria D, Fragaa S, Braun KO, Unfer B.

Behavior of the elderly with regard to hygiene procedures for and maintenance of removable dentures.

Oral Health Prev Dent 2016;14:21-26.

25. Deniz DA, Kulak Ozkan Y.

The influence of occlusion on masticatory performance and satisfaction in complete denture wearers.

J Oral Rehabil. 2013;40(2):91-8.

26. Devaki VN, Balu K, Ramesh SB, Arvind RJ, Venkatesan.

Pre-prosthetic surgery: Mandible.

J Pharm Bioall Sci 2012;4:414-6.

27. Dostálová T, Radina P, Seydlová M, Zvárová J, Valenta Z.
Overdenture – Implants versus Teeth – Quality of Life and Objective Therapy Evaluation.
Prague Medical Report 2009;110:332–342.

28. Fajri L, Benfdil F, Abdelkoui A, Merzouk N.
Contribution of tissue conditioning to increasing the mandibular support surface in complete removable dentures: A clinical case report.
Web Journal du Dentiste December 2016;10:11-20.

29. Fajri L, Benfdil F, El Mohtarim B, El Wady W, Abdedine A. Complete mandibular prostheses: stability and retention. *Actual Odonto-Stomatol 2009;247:267-86.*

30. Fajri L, Benfdil F, Merzouk N, El Mohtarim B, Abdedine A.
Diagnosis and management of prosthetic-related mucosal lesions in completely edentulous patients.
Actual Odonto-Stomatol 2008;243:225-238.

31. Fajri L, Berrada S, AbdedineA.
Clinical examination contributing to selection and orientation of prosthodontic treatments in completely edentulous patients.
Rev Odont Stomat 2008;37:91-107

32. Feine JS, Carlsson GE, Awad MA et al.
The McGill Consensus Statement on Overdentures. Mandibular two-implant overdentures as first choice standard of care for edentulous patients.
Gerodontology 2002;19(1):3-4.

33. Felton D, Cooper L, Duqum I et al.
Evidence-Based Guidelines for the Care and Maintenance of Complete Dentures: A Publication of the American College of Prosthodontists.
Journal of Prosthodontics 2011;20: S1–S12.

34. Genin G.
The orientation of the mandibular occlusal plane in complete removable prostheses: from complex to everyday practice [thesis].

Nancy: Faculty of Dental Surgery, Nancy, 2012.

35. Guessous DF, Regragui A, Merzouk N, Benfdil F.

How to ensure prosthetic stability in conventional complete removable dentures (CRPD)?

Actual Odonto-Stomatol 2018;289:p5.

36. Gueye M, Mbodj E B, Dieng L, Tchibozo G, Touré A, Thioune N.

Remodeling of stabilizing polished surfaces in complete removable prostheses: a clinical case report.

Rev Col Odonto-Stomatol Afr Chir Maxillo-fac, 2015;22(2):5-9.

37. Hasnaoui Y.

Pre-prosthetic surgery in the totally edentulous patient for complete removable bimaxillary prostheses [thesis].

Nancy: Faculty of Dentistry, 2017.

38. Hauteville A, Cohen A.S.

Manual of Surgical Dentistry.

Paris: Masson; 1989. Chapter 9.

39. Helfer M, Louis JP, Vermande G.

Management of intermaxillary relationships in complete removable prostheses.

Prosthetic Strategy 2010;10(1):33-41.

40. Huard C, Bessadet M, Jalabert-Malbos ML et al.

The contribution of mini-implants in the treatment of total mandibular edentulism.

Actual Odonto-Stomatol 2011;256:305-313

41. Huard C, Bessadet M, Nicolas E, Veyrune J L.

Geriatric slim implants for complete denture wearers: clinical aspects and perspectives.

Clin Cosmet Investig Dent. 2013;5:63–68.

42. Hue O, Berteretche MV.

Complete dentures: is tissue conditioning still relevant?

Actual Odonto-Stomatol 2014;268:24-28.

43. Hue O, Berteretche MV.

Complete dentures: clinical reality and therapeutic solutions.

Paris: Quintessance International, 2003.

44. Hue O.

Polished stabilizing surfaces in partial dentures.

LQOS 1982;25:323-344.

45. Itic A.

Some keys to successful complete mandibular prostheses.

Prosthetic Strategy 2018;2:111-121.

46. Kimoto S, Kimoto K, Gunji A, Kawai Y, Murakami H, Tanaka K, et al.

(Clinical effects of acrylic resilient denture liners applied to mandibular complete dentures on the alveolar ridge.

J Oral Rehabil. Nov 2007;34(11):862-9.

47. Klein P.

Some definitions to better understand piezography.

Inf Dent 1989;71(29):2519-23

48. Koronis S, Pizatos E, Polyzois G, Lagouvardos P.

Clinical evaluation of three denture cushion adhesives by complete denture wearers.

Gerodontology 2012;29: e161–e169

49. Kutkut A, Bertoli E, Frazer R, Pinto-Sinai G, Hidalgo RF, Studt J.

A systematic review of studies comparing conventional complete dentures and implant-retained overdentures.

Journal of prosthodontic research 2018;62(1):1–9

50. Lamrous F., & Nabid A.

Modeling the optimal prosthetic space: which function to use?

Strat Prothétique. June 2015;15(3):169-80.

51. Lejoyeux J, Lejoyeux R.

Tissue conditioning in removable prostheses.

Paris: Masson; 1993.

52. Lejoyeux J.

Tissue conditioning.

RFOS 1962.

53. Lejoyeux J.

Complete Prosthesis Volume 1.
Published by Librairie Maloine, Paris, 1973.

54. Lejoyeux J.
Treatment of Total Edentulism: Third-Year Course.
Ed. Maloine 1986.

55. Makzoume JE.
Morphologic comparison of two neutral zone impression techniques: A pilot study.
J Prosthet Dent 2004;92:563-8.

56. Mellinger G.
The value of implants in complete removable prostheses: current concepts and guide to surgical and prosthetic implementation [thesis].
Nancy: Faculty of Dentistry, 2011.

57. Mersel A.
Piezographic solution for class III bimaxillary edentulism.
Conference at the Garancière talks, Paris, 1984

58. Millet C, Fournier J.
3 Implant-retained complete removable prosthesis.

59. Munoz CA, Gendreau L, Shanga G, Magnuszewski T, Fernandez P, Duroche J. (69)
A Clinical Study to Evaluate Denture Adhesive Use in Well-Fitting Dentures.
Journal of Prosthodontics: Implant, Esthetic and Reconstructive Dentistry 2012;21(2):123–129.

60. Papadiochou S, Emmanouil I, Papadiochos I.
Adhesive dentures: A systematic review.
The Journal of prosthetic dentistry 2015;113(5):391-397.

61. Park JH, Lee JY, Sang-Wan Shin SW.
Treatment Outcomes for Mandibular Mini-Implant–Retained Overdentures: A Systematic Review.
Int J Prosthodont 2017;30:269–276.

62. Perez C, D'Incau E, DupuisV.
Improving the stability of complete mandibular dentures.

Alternatives 2004;24:39-46.

63. **Porwal A, Sasaki K.**

Current status of the neutral zone: A literature review.

J Prosthet Dent 2013;109:129-134.

64. **Postaire M, Daas M, Dada K.**

Prostheses and implants for the completely edentulous mandible.

Quintessence International, Paris, 2006.

65. **Regragui A, Abdedine A, Merzouk N.**

Biofunctional space and tissue conditioning: what are the prospects for complete removable prostheses?

Actual Odonto-Stomatol 2011;255:197-206.

66. **Regragui A, Benfdil F, Abdedine A.**

The value of stabilizing polished surfaces in the management of a complex case of complete removable prostheses.

Actual Odonto-Stomatol 2010;249:43-58.

67. **Regragui A, Sefrioui A, Berrada S, Merzouk N.**

Buccal bone hypertrophy in the completely edentulous: a fatality to be avoided!

Actual Odonto-Stomatol 2016;275:2.

68. **Rehmann P, Künkel AK, Weber D, Lotzmann U, Wöstmann B.** Using a Modified Neutral Zone Technique to Improve the Stability of Mandibular Complete Dentures: A Prospective Clinical Study.

Int J Prosthodont 2016;29:570–572.

69. **Rehmann P, Zenginel M, Wöstmann B.**

Alternative Procedure to Improve the Stability of Mandibular Complete Dentures: A Modified Neutral Zone Technique

Int J Prosthodont 2012;25:506–508.

70. **Rignon-Bret C, Rignon-Bret JM.**

Complete removable prosthesis—immediate prosthesis—supraradicular and implant-supported prosthesis.

Paris: CdP, 2002.

71. **Rignon-Bret C.**

Attachments and complete supra-radicular and supra-implant prostheses.
Paris, Edition cahier de prothèse, 2008.

72. Rokhssi H, Abdelkoui A, Merzouk N, Benfdil F. Piezographic impressions in everyday practice. *Actual Odonto-Stomatol 2018;289:3*

73. Saadi N.
Improvement of insufficient support surfaces for prosthetic balance [thesis].
Monastir: Faculty of Dental Medicine, Monastir, 2016

74. Shah FK, Gebreel A, Elshokouki AH, Habib AA, Porwal A. Comparison of immediate complete denture, tooth and implant-supported overdenture on vertical dimension and muscle activity.
J Adv Prosthoont 2012;4:61-71.

75. Stephan G, Noharet R, Mariani P.
Choice of occlusal concept in totally edentulous patients rehabilitated with implant-supported prostheses.
Prosthetic Strategy 2006;6(1):35-46.

76. Stromberg WR, Hickey JC.
Comparison of physiologically and manually formed denture bases.
J Prosthet Dent 1965;15:213-30.

77. Susset M.
Complete removable supra-radicular versus supra-implant mandibular prosthesis [Thesis].
Nantes: Nantes Dentistry Training and Research Unit, 2015.

78. Sutton AF, & McCord JF.
A randomized clinical trial comparing anatomic, lingualized, and zero-degree posterior occlusal forms for complete dentures.
J Prosthet Dent. May 2007;97(5):292-8.

79. Thomas J
Treatment of Edentulism: Optimizing Outcomes with Tissue Management and Impression Techniques.
Journal of Prosthodontics: Implant, Esthetic and Reconstructive Dentistry, 2009;18(2):97-105.

80. Toquet T, Briot M, Exbrayat P.
The mandibular supra-implant complete denture: current data and protocol for fabrication.
Le fil dentaire 2009;44:26-30.

81. Tosello A, Chevaux JM.
Repair of prosthetic bases.
Encycl Méd Chir, Odontologie, 23-325-H-10, 2001, 8 p.

82. Triki M.
Complete removable supra-radicular versus supra-implant mandibular prosthesis [thesis].
Monastir: Faculty of Dental Medicine of Monastir, 2018.

83. Warreth A, Alkadhimi AF, Sultan A, Byrne C, Woods E.
Mandibular implant-supported overdentures: attachment systems, and number and locations of implants - Part I.
Journal of the Irish Dental Association 2015;61(2):93-97.

84. Warreth A, Alkadhimi AF, Sultan A, Byrne C, Woods E.
Mandibular implant-supported overdentures: attachment systems, and number and locations of implants - Part II.
Journal of the Irish Dental Association 2015;61(3):144-148.

85. Wong A.
Single-implant-supported complete mandibular prosthesis: a literature review [thesis].
Bordeaux: College of Health Sciences, 2018.

Internet references

86. Charrier M, De Valbray R.

Stabilized supra-implant prosthesis: criteria for choosing attachment systems.

[Accessed on 5/10/2020], available at the following URL:

https://www.lefildentaire.com/articles/clinique/implantologie/prothese-supra-implantaire-stabilisee-criteres-de-choix-des-systemes-dattachement/#:~:text=Les%20implants%20supportant%20les%20syst%C3%A8mes,en%20cas%20de%20forces%20parasites

87. Gardon-Mollard G.

PACSI: What implant positioning?

[Accessed on 5/10/2020], available at the URL: https://www.idweblogs.com/e-implanto-proth/pacsi-quel-positionnement- implantaire/

88. Guessous F et al.

Piezography: the technique of choice for treating flat and negative mandibular ridges #1

[Accessed on 5/10/2020], available at: https://www.idweblogs.com/edentement-total/piezographie%E2%80%89- technique-de-choix-dans-la-prise-en-charge-des-cretes-plates-et-negatives-mandibulaires-1/

Kolibri 360 GmbH
Ferdinand-Jühlke-Straße 7
99095 Erfurt, Deutschland
produktsicherheit@kolibri360.de

Druck:
CPI Druckdienstleistungen GmbH
im Auftrag der
Kolibri 360 GmbH
Ferdinand-Jühlke-Str. 7
99095 Erfurt